PEAC
THE ESSENTIAL (

The most comprehensive and practical chronicle of accompanying I have read. The emotional information is often missing in other publications but was covered here with such truth and love. The pictures and journal at the end made the telling personal and the love expressed so real. In reading the journal all the practical advice was integrated with real daily events.

Evelyn Newton, RN CHPN, Director of Patient Services
Highway Christian Hospice, www.home.earthlink.net/~hch1996

Simply and compassionately addresses everything you need to know to care for your loved one on their final journey. From the very beginning to the very end and beyond, it guides you in making decisions, how to provide care, dealing with emotions and spirituality and everything else to expect on the way. Not only a resource to help care for the dying but help to find the strength and peace to live on.

Sharon Criscione, RN,BSN,CHPN, Clinical Director
The Martin and Edith Stein Hospice, www.wilfcampus.org/steinhospice

A wonderful guide for caregivers during the dying process. The educational benefit to family members with a dying loved one at home is phenomenal. The author has used her own experiences to prepare families for each step of the journey. I thought the exercises at the end of each chapter were a great start to the bereavement process.

Kim Shaw, RN, CHPN, CHPCA, Vice-President
Sojourn Care of Arizona, www.sojourncare.com

This was written with truth, love, compassion and caring by someone who has had to make the difficult choices concerning her loved one. It is an excellent resource for all those who must face this end-of-life journey.

Fr. Tony Carillo, Hospice Chaplain
Hospice Inspiris, www.hospiceinspiris.com

Very practical and informative, with a true-life, heartfelt ending. Families will benefit from the information in this book.

Susan Meyer, RN, Director of Clinical Services
Grace Hospice, www.gracehospice.org

This book holds such honest, loving insight into caring for a loved one on their final journey. Simple, practical, and a wealth of knowledge ... it truly is a safe harbor for the unique gift of walking someone home.

Jane McElroy, RN
NJ Hospice & Palliative Care Org., www.njhospice.org

An exceptional tool and resource for anyone assisting or witnessing a loved one going through their final journey. It is a delightful, heartfelt, open discussion of processes, tips and things to ponder when traveling with them. Well done, and I applaud you. Thank you from all of us.

JoAnne Simonian, Director of Nursing
The Crossing Hospice Care, www.hrcaz.com/go2/crossings-hospice.cfm

---

Thank God for a resource that deals with the difficult issues so that we, and those for whom we care, can make a Peaceful Passage. Navigating through the rough waters, West addresses common fears and sometimes unresolved emotional issues, all the while working through the struggles around faith and God. This book is essential in bringing life to loved ones and caregivers, preparing everyone for the spiritual, emotional and psychological journey ahead.

Steve Drennan, Chaplain and Bereavement Coordinator
Affinity Hospice of Life, www.affinityhospice.com

It is obvious this was written by someone who has firsthand experience traveling this journey and a heart to share it with others. Practical, useful, and presented in a compassionate, caring, and gentle way, not only is the book informative but is an interesting, enjoyable read. I recommend everyone taking this journey to read the book.

Linda S. Segrest, RN, CHPN, Director of Hospice Services
Baptist Health, www.baptistfirst.org

Very insightful and informative. It would be a blessing to have this book at the bedside of a loved one regardless if they are in a Hospice environment or being taken care of by the family. The emotional and physical experiences shared would feel common to others as they attempt to understand what is "normal" and what may come next.

Terry A. Baxter, Chaplain
Hearts for Hospice, www.heartsforhospice.com

The author takes the reader on a comforting journey as she parallels her personal experience as witness to the death of her mother, to the journey we all experience during that end phase of life. The reader will find peace as a result of their increased understanding of the events leading to death.

Royle D. Schmidt, RN, General Manager
Hospice Family Care, Inc., www.hfc-az.com

The book has a lot of useful information for people searching to learn about hospice. It gives information to help the patient and the caregiver along this path.

Kaye Maxwell, Administrator
Chattahoochee Hospice, www.chattahoocheehospice.com

Well-written, easy-to-understand and full of valuable and vital information for end of life needs. The author shares her own story, making the words even more meaningful. She easily navigates the waters of caring for a dying person in a dignified and compassionate way. This book will, no doubt, become a solid resource to persons taking care of those they love in their final days.

Lisa Hanne RN, Administrator
Sun Valley Hospice, www.sunvalleyhospice.com

A tremendous help in identifying needs and expectations as one begins the journey as a caregiver. Expect helpful hints in many areas including finding a hospice, marriage, family, work and faith issues. A wonderful guide providing comfort from the help the book offers.

Patty Baggett, RN, BSN, BC, CSD
Hospice Advantage/EAMC, www.hospiceadvantage.com

The author embraces the philosophy and spirituality of bringing honor and affirmation to one's life during its final stages. Accurate, easy to understand, and an excellent, comprehensive guide for anyone facing the death of a loved one.

Paula Wolf-Bellias, RN LNC, Quality Assurance / Performance Improvement coordinator
Compassionate Care Hospice (New Jersey office) www.cchnet.net

Unlike most books of this type which are either information or personal experience, Kim has done a great job of combining the two to give the reader a resource on both levels. She has done an excellent job of showing what hospice is about - not helping someone die, but helping them live until they die.

Julia Campbell, RN, Patient Care Administrator
Hospice of the Southwest, www.hospiceofthesouthwest.com

This compassion-driven book makes the journey of caring at home vivid and real, as if it were happening to the reader right now. West achieves this through her exhaustive practical detail (such as the kind and quantity of bed linens needed, how to wash the loved one's hair in bed, and what kinds of food to aim for and which to avoid). She also achieves this, especially on the emotional and spiritual levels, through allowing us the privilege of seeing her diary of what her journey was like. Even for myself, a seasoned hospice chaplain, I was deeply moved by its authenticity.

Rabbi Karen Bookman Kaplan, Board Certified Hospice Chaplain
Princeton Homecare Services, www.princetonhcs.org

I wish I had had this step-by-step journey when my father and my mother, three years apart departed this world. As a professional working in an environment of respite and palliative care for children the thought process on what is important in life has a whole new set of priorities. A good read filled with important messages, thank you.

Kim Knotter, Director of Development
Ryan House, www.ryanhouse.org

Peaceful Passage

The essential guide to navigating the emotional storms and daily logistics of an at-home end-of-life journey

Kim West, PhD

New Heart Publishing, Phoenix, Arizona
2011

This book includes information from many sources and personal experience. It is published for general reference and is not intended to be a substitute for independent verification by readers when necessary and appropriate. The book is sold with the understanding that neither the author nor publisher is engaged in rendering any legal, psychological or medical advice. The publisher and author disclaim any personal liability, directly or indirectly, for advice or information presented within. Although the author and publisher have prepared this manuscript with utmost care and diligence and have made every effort to ensure the accuracy and completeness of the information contained within, we assume no responsibility for errors, inaccuracies, omissions or inconsistencies.

Publisher's Cataloging-in-Publication

West, Kim, 1955-

Peaceful passage : the essential guide to navigating the emotional storms and daily logistics of an at-home end-of-life journey / Kim West. -- 1st ed.

p. cm.

Includes index.

LCCN 2010904523

ISBN-13: 978-0-9840526-6-0

ISBN-10: 0-9840526-6-6

1. Terminal care--Psychological aspects. 2. Terminally ill. 3. Caregivers. 4. Home care services. I. Title.

R726.8.W47 2011 362.17'5

QBI10-600076

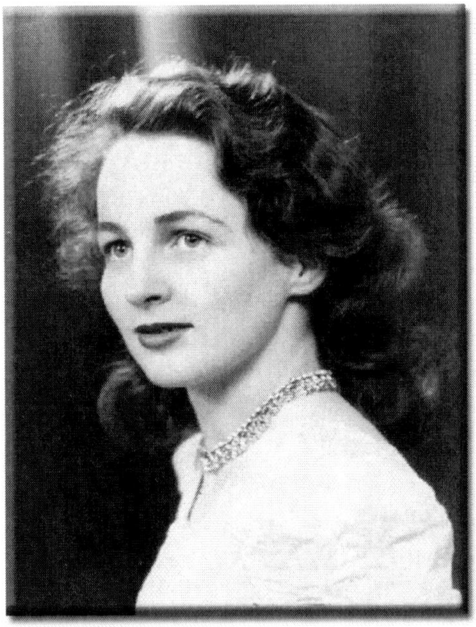

Helen Terese Sullivan
January 5, 1931 - July 10, 2009

Table of Contents

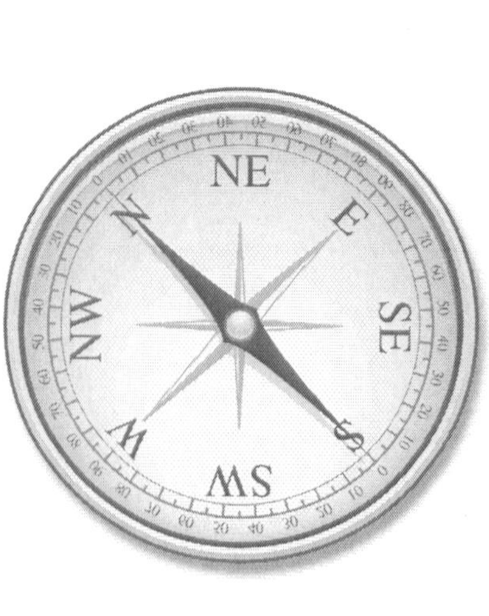
NE
N
E
SE

Introduction

I looked down at Mom lying there unconscious. The hospice nurse was trying to take Mom's blood pressure, but it wasn't registering. Hand to my mouth, tears slowly moving down my face I looked at the nurse helplessly. She walked around the bed, put her arm around me and said, "Kim, this is what we have been working so hard for." The concept startled me. "Really? Have I been working toward her death? Is that what I have been doing?"

Caring for a dying loved one is an extraordinary experience and an amazing privilege. It is also a journey with a known destination that we deny right up until we reach its shores. We know it is coming and are surprised when it actually arrives. We long for it to be over and dread that it actually will. It is a sacred, amazing and, sometimes frightening passage.

And, now, you are about to take this journey with your loved one.

I'M SORRY YOU ARE HOLDING THIS BOOK

It means that someone you love is dying and that you are about to enter a trying season of life that may be harder than you imagine. You might be truly frightened about what is to come or maybe you only need some guidance and encouragement. Either way, I want to help you through this time.

By giving you a map, a compass and a lot of encouragement, I hope to help make this a more peaceful passage for you and your loved one. This essential guide will facilitate that process.

I'M GLAD YOU ARE HOLDING THIS BOOK

You are entering a time of personal growth that may be unlike anything you have been through before. You will be challenged to reevaluate yourself and your beliefs and you will find resources inside you that you didn't know were there.

There will be days when you are filled with energy and love. There will also be days when you are exhausted physically, emotionally, mentally and spiritually. I want you to know that...

...You are stronger than you think you are.

...You are more courageous than you think you can be.

...You are able to take this journey.

...You are not going through this alone.

THIS BOOK IS YOUR GUIDE FOR THE JOURNEY

It is designed for the time after the decision for hospice has been made. It will show you how to pick the right help, how to care for your loved one, what to expect, the emotional changes you will both experience, and techniques to help you handle these changes well.

It will help you cope with the emotional storms while giving you practical, hands-on knowledge to care for your loved one, giving you answers for some of your questions and resources to find others.

We will talk about family and friends, finances and hands-on care-giving, children and grief, as well as much more. You can keep this book as a handy resource as you move from the beginning to the end of this journey.

You will find checklists to keep you organized and pages for you to chronicle your own journey. The book is designed so that you can quickly and easily find the information you need.

Our goal here is to keep you on course, guide your daily life and not let you get shipwrecked on the way.

I encourage you to journal, either in the pages in this book or elsewhere. This journey's log is something you will return to many times and read. It will recount this amazing time in your life and be a treasure to you later in life.

So, I know you have a lot of questions and a lot to do. Let's get started.

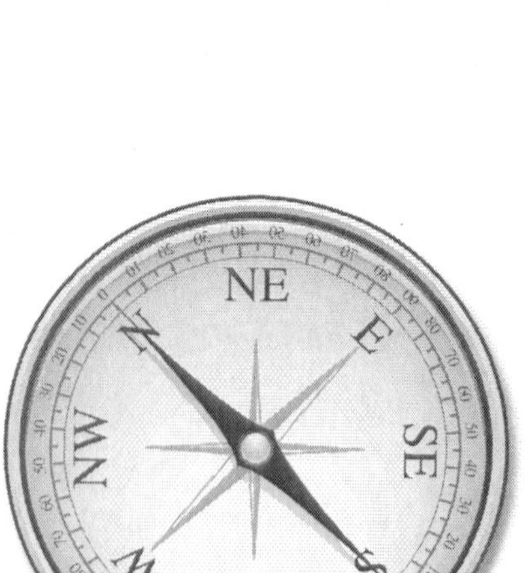
NE
E
SE

Chapter One

THE JOURNEY BEFORE YOU

It is not down in any map; true places never are.

~Herman Melville

HEARING THE NEWS THAT A CURE IS NO LONGER POSSIBLE

The car accident was the first indication that something was wrong with Mom. Testing showed that she had a brain tumor. Further testing showed a tumor on her pancreas as well. Both of these are fatal for a 78-year-old woman.

We talked with specialists. We did our research on the net, and we all came to the conclusion that what was best was to allow Mom to have a good quality of life for the time she had left: statistically 40-80 days.

This news that Mom was dying came on us suddenly. For you, this news may have come over a period of time, perhaps a lengthy illness. Regardless of the delivery, we always seem unprepared for the final prognosis.

YOUR FIRST REACTIONS TO THE NEWS

Shock and numbness often arrive first, followed quickly by denial. Could this really be true? Maybe the tests are wrong. It seems like a bad dream and at first we walk around stunned. It is surreal. We wonder, "What will come next and what should I do next?"

After the initial shock wears off, we must begin planning for the journey. Much as we would like to, there is no way to avoid these life transitions. We, and those we love, will all come to this final passage and, so, preparations must be made. You can meet this journey determined to be prepared and travel it well. You have the power to do so even though you might not know this yet. At this time of great stress and sorrow you can become the best version of yourself, the strongest, and most resilient you. You probably just need some help and encouragement and someone to stay beside you throughout the journey. I will stay with you through these pages.

THIS IS A FAMILY MATTER

In most circumstances, you will be working with your family as your loved one enters this journey. There are different ways to arrive at the same destination and others may have different routes in mind than you. Sometimes the plans that need to be made are done so with many voices inputing their thoughts and desires. And some of them are conflicting.

You are already dealing with your and your loved one's emotions and now you will also be exposed to the emotions of family and friends. Not all of them will respond well. If your relationships are not healthy and up to date then you might want to anticipate any potential emotional unrest as you head into this situation.

Remember that your family members are experiencing their own denial and grief emotions, and will be processing them out loud and in their actions. Keeping this in mind will help you as you work with them.

Begin by explaining the information and medical actions that have led to this decision for an at-home end-of-life journey. Some family members may want to fight for more treatment, seek other opinions, or simply not accept the loved one's decision to die peacefully at home. If your loved one is present and capable, have them directly discuss their wishes for their end of life. If your loved one is not present speak for them, being careful not to speak from your own wishes but accurately representing what your loved one has told you or what is in place in their advance directives.

Some may want to take over and dictate what is to happen next. There may be financial arguments. Others may be grief-stricken and want you to care for them too. Remember, everyone is going through this in their own way and it may not be your way. What is needed is patience, good communication and that everyone has the opportunity to speak their mind and state their preferences.

WHAT DOES YOUR LOVED ONE WANT?

Before any decisions are made, you must first approach your loved one. This is *their* journey on which you are privileged to accompany them. What do they want? Finding out their wishes affirms their dignity and ensures that they will be treated with the utmost respect.

Ask your loved one **who they want to make health care decisions** for them when they cannot act on their own behalf. The person they choose will oversee their care, handle interactions with hospice and Medicare and provide that they are in the right place and have the right staff to care for them when they need it most.

Find out the kind of **medical interventions** they want and do not want: your loved one has the right to have or not have life-enhancing or life sustaining intervention. These advance directives guarantee that your loved one will not receive or have withheld care that they desire.

How do they want to be cared for? This care includes how they want the pain managed (should it arise), their wishes for spiritual support, and their personal hygiene guidelines.

How do they want to be treated? Do they prefer being touched? Do they want to be prayed for? To die at home? To be with people? To be alone? Remember, it is their decision how they will be treated.

What do they want others to know? Do they wish to keep personal information personal? Do they want others to know their spiritual beliefs and how that is impacting their journey? How do they want to be remembered? What are their personal wishes for family members? How do they want their remains are to be treated?

Talking about charting the course will be a difficult conversation but as you work together, you can come to an agreement where your loved one's wishes are honored and everyone is heard.

In these conversations, you will need to make short and long term goals, divide the responsibilities where you can (more on this in Chapter Five), and decide who will be the primary caregiver if your loved one has not specified.

There are also some tougher decisions to make.

A MAP OF POSSIBLE INTERVENTIONS AND MEDICATIONS

There are things you and your loved one need to decide now regarding medical interventions and medications. Thinking through the possibilities now is essential for this journey. Your ability to make decisions is going to be clouded by emotion and exhaustion as time progresses. Remember that you can change your mind later if you need to, for now, you are saying this is what we think is best.

As you think through the different medical interventions and medications that you might have to choose, keep in mind that the goal is to make your loved one's end-of-life journey comfortable and not to simply prolong their life. You want them to have a good quality of life, not just extend it.

Discuss all of these decisions in detail with your hospice team. Ask questions so that you can make the best-informed decision for your loved one. The hospice professionals are there to help you with these tough choices and will provide you with support as you do.

Artificial feeding and hydration: These can be helpful as a temporary measure but should not be thought of as life-extending. As the body moves closer to death, it will need less food and water. For those of us watching, that can be a bit frightening. While we don't want our loved one to suffer, there isn't any indication that the body wanting less food is painful or even uncomfortable.

When water cannot be given by mouth, some family members might want an IV (intravenous fluid) started. An IV can also administer pain medications, but most times pain meds can be given in other ways. However, IV fluids can also cause congestive heart problems and lead to fluid build up in the lungs—causing the very discomfort you are trying to avoid. Using an IV for dehydration might help with symptoms such as shaking or confusion, but can also cause swelling and prolong suffering.

A feeding tube is sometimes wanted by those caring for their loved one when food is no longer wanted or tolerated. As the body dies it needs little food and force feeding will not stop the coming death. What your loved one has stated they want and speaking in depth with your hospice team will help you make a decision for or against artificial feeding.

Oxygen: Giving oxygen can be helpful to ease anxiety when shortness of breath is present. Deciding to use oxygen is about bringing comfort not about extending life.

Antibiotics: If there is an infection that is secondary to the disease, antibiotics may be desired. However, there are some instances in which the antibiotic may prolong your loved one's suffering. For example, pneumonia used to be called, "an old man's best friend" because it allowed the dying to just fall asleep and drift away. By using antibiotics you might unnecessarily prolong death and suffering.

DNR/CPR: A decision to use hospice doesn't mean you must have a DNR (do not resuscitate) order and Medicare prohibits disqualification based on this status. However, being on hospice means that your loved one is dying and resuscitation may only prolong discomfort. Hospice will work with you to understand the benefits and burdens of all options and will support you whatever you choose.

Pain control: If pain is present you and your loved one will want to find relief from it. We will talk about pain medications later in the book but here you want to talk about what your loved one wants. Some pain medications can cause your loved one to sleep a great deal of the time and lose time to interact with the family. Ask your loved one if s/he would rather be pain free but asleep or have some discomfort but be awake to interact.

These decisions on care are made based on your loved one's wishes and a family discussion of care options. Make sure you understand them and ask questions until you do. Making informed choices brings peace to those decisions and keeps you from questioning yourself later. These choices need to be put into writing and they are called, "Advance Directives."

FINANCIAL AND LEGAL MATTERS

Advance Directives: This is a document that will give instructions on what is or is not to be done in health care if a person becomes unable to make medical decisions. It usually includes a Living Will, Medical Power of Attorney, and any other needed directives. This needs to be signed in front of a Notary with two witnesses unrelated to the loved one and with no interest in their estate.

Even if your loved one has put these wishes in writing, family members may try to fight for or against certain treatments. Nonetheless, having advance directives in place and your loved one's wishes spoken and written will be of big help here to ensure their wishes are carried out.

Power of Attorney for medical purposes: This document names one person that can make decisions as an agent for the ill person. This person will decide on treatment (or withholding treatment) on the patient's behalf. This is a very important person and one that must be trusted to act in the best interests and same intent as the person who is ill.

If there is not a will, power of attorney for medical and financial decisions and advance directives in place then this needs to be a priority to be completed before your loved one deteriorates too far. Having this in place creates boundaries for their care and for their possessions.

Will: This document is essential. Without a will, the journey for the family members after the loved one has passed can be both long and frustrating. The will lays out your loved one's wishes for disposal of their possessions and estate after they pass. It ensures an easy transition and can keep problems in the family from arising.

Power of Attorney: The individual named to have power to make financial and legal decisions can be the person named as executor of the will or someone else. This individual is responsible for paying all debts and liabilities while the loved one is ill and gives them the power to carry out the loved one's financial wishes.

My sister and I shared ***Medical*** *Power of Attorney. This meant that either of us could make medical decisions for our mother. As we live in different states, it was good to be able to make medical decisions quickly and on my own for our mother when she was in my home. When she had an infection I could decide on antibiotics, when she fell out of bed in the middle of the night and was injured I was able to get medical care for her without calling and waking my sister.*

We held Power of Attorney together for my mother's estate, and, unlike the Medical Power of Attorney we had to make all these decision together. This meant that both of us had to sign any legal documents that dealt directly with personal property, bank accounts, etc. This made some things more difficult, as we had to send documents back and forth so we could both sign them and we had to go to her banks together, but it was not a major problem.

It is important to provide copies of the needed paperwork to everyone involved. Transparency helps to keep the lines of communication open and clear.

THIS IS ABOUT THEM

Your loved one is important by essence of their very existence. Every human has that dignity and should be treated this way no matter what is happening to them physically. Treat them as a living breathing human being until the moment they die.

The goal is to ensure a peaceful passage. In order to do so you will need additional help.

CHAPTER ONE WORKBOOK

WHAT DOES YOUR LOVED ONE WANT?

Personal care

- Spiritual support? ______________________________

- Personal hygiene? ______________________________

- Touched or not? ______________________________

- Prayed for? ______________________________

- To die at home? ______________________________

- To be with people? To be alone? ______________________________

Others to know about

- Personal information or about the illness? ____________

____

____

____

- Spiritual beliefs and how that is impacting their journey?

____

____

____

- How they want to be remembered? ____________

____

____

____

- Their personal wishes for family members? ____________

____

____

____

- How they want their remains are to be treated? ______

____

____

____

Who will have Medical Power of Attorney? ____________

____

____

____

How has the family delegated responsibilities? ____________

____

____

____

Decisions on interventions:

- Artificial feeding and hydration ______________________
- Oxygen ______________________
- Antibiotics ______________________
- Pain control ______________________
- Additional treatments ______________________

JOURNAL

When I first head the news...

What I feel about:

- Family involvements ______________________________

- Medical decisions ______________________________

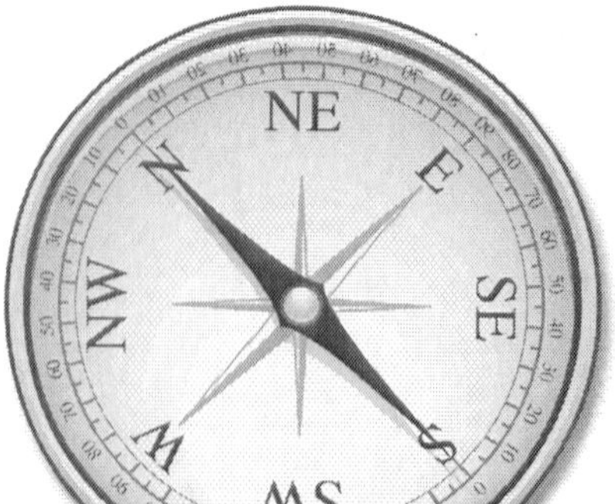

Chapter Two

CHARTING A COURSE

A person often meets his destiny on the road he took to avoid it.

~Jean de La Fontaine

HOSPICE WILL TAKE THIS JOURNEY WITH YOU

The decision has been made to start on this journey. You have talked this over with your loved one and family, and, now, you will need help. Your doctor will refer you to hospice for that help.

A person usually turns to hospice in the last six months of their life, but it can be longer. Some people even leave hospice for a time if they seem improved. (They can come back on it later if needed.)

When enrolled in hospice, the attention turns from frantic and aggressive medical treatment to love and comfort care. The goal for the duration of the journey is to bring reassurance, support, and nurture for the loved one who is dying as well as to the family.

PICK THE RIGHT CREW FOR THE JOURNEY

There are over 5000 hospice organizations in the United States, and—although they all have the same goal of comfort care—they may have a different feel or competency level.

To pick a hospice, first choose two or three. Look at their web sites to get a good idea of what a particular hospice is like. Are they large or small organizations? Do they seem very business-like or very soft and supportive? One type is not better than another and the choice is really up to your preference. If you want a very structured, organized type of help then choose that. If you want something more gentle and laid-back but still competent then choose that type of hospice.

Be careful to pick the right hospice for you and your loved one. They will be involved in helping you at a time that is intimate and sensitive. They will need to provide detailed attention and competency while not adding to your anxiety.

If you do choose a hospice organization that does not seem to be compatible, you can change hospices once a benefit periord. You have enough on your plate without having to struggle with your hospice care. If you need to change, do so. Your new hospice will be happy to help you with the transition.

BENEFITS YOUR LOVED ONE IS ENTITLED TO THROUGH HOSPICE

- Nursing support and care
- Medical equipment and supplies
- Medications related to the diagnosis
- Social services and counseling
- Nursing assistant services

WHO PAYS FOR IT?

Hospice is paid for in a variety of methods including Medicare, Medicaid (in most states) and many private health insurance plans. If your loved one is not eligible for Medicare and has no insurance, you may still be able to get hospice help. A Medicare-certified hospice will provide hospice care to everyone who is eligible regardless of their ability to pay. Don't assume your loved one qualifies or doesn't qualify. Call your chosen hospice and ask for an evaluation. They will be happy to make calls on your behalf to determine your loved one's eligibility and qualification.

LEVELS OF HOSPICE CARE

Routine care: Intermittent visits at home each week. This is the most common type of care.

Inpatient care: Provided on a short-term basis to manage symptoms. This cannot be used for tests or treatment toward a cure. These centers usually have a home-like feel to them and your loved one will receive skilled nursing care until their symptoms have stabilized and they can return home.

Respite care: Available occasionally up to five consecutive days at a time. Your loved one would be transferred to an inpatient care facility for those five days so that you can rest and renew.

Continuous care: Provided in the home on a short-term basis during a crisis. Sometimes a person needs something between routine and inpatient care. Hospice might then decide to have someone stay in the home for a short time to care for your loved one and manage their symptoms.

THE HOSPICE TEAM

Doctor supervisor: You may never see this doctor but s/he is in constant contact with the nurse supervisor. S/he will advise on care and medications and be available for questions. Every time a nurse visits, they will relay all your loved one's vital statistics, a description of how they are doing, and questions for continued care to this doctor. The doctor supervises the care, writes prescriptions, and places new care orders.

Nurse: Usually, you will be assigned two nurses—one of whom will supervise the care team. They will visit 1-3 times per week, check medications, and order them for you as needed. They are also available to answer questions and to teach how to give care and give personal support.

CNA: This person is a Certified Nursing Assistant and will come 1-3 times per week to help with personal care and grooming. A good CNA will make a world of difference for you and your loved one. They carefully and with great skill perform hands-on care-giving and can teach you good tips that you can use immediately.

Social worker: A social worker will help with benefits, counseling, grief, and funeral resources. You may or may not need their help to a great extent, but they are available to you.

Physical and occupational therapist: As mobility is lost, this person will assist you in teaching you positioning as well as how to move and care for your loved one.

Chaplain: The chaplain will come as requested to provide spiritual support for your loved one and the family.

Volunteers: These people will not provide care but are available to sit with and talk with your loved one. In the meantime, you can run errands or take a much needed break.

WHAT TO EXPECT FROM THE TEAM

The team will ask what you and your loved one want and help set goals for the best care and comfort. They will meet at least every two weeks to discuss your loved one's progress and make sure the goals are being met. The Primary Physician can still participate in care and remain informed by the hospice case manager.

You can expect help 24-hours-a-day when needed. A 3 am crisis phone call will bring a helpful voice and immediate assistance. A nurse will come to your home when needed, no matter the time or the day. Often, they can offer you comforting help directly over the phone.

They will bring comfort care to your loved one but will not attempt to prolong life. When difficult symptoms arise, they will do all in their power to alleviate the pain and restore a level of comfort. They are experts on which medications and therapies to use and will continue to work to find the right combinations of medications to eliminate pain or discomfort.

They will answer questions, educate you on the disease and the process, explain caring techniques, and suggest medical equipment and medications. If you need a hug, they can do that, too.

They will treat your loved one as the person they are and not the disease they have. You can expect respect, care, concern, and dignity.

They are there to help your loved one, you, and your family as you work through emotional issues and grief. They will continue to be there for you a year after your loved one has completed their passage.

CHAPTER TWO WORKBOOK

CHOOSING YOUR HOSPICE

Your doctor may have referred you to a particular hospice. Just know that you can pick your own. A quick web search will bring up the hospices in your area. Look over their sites and get a feel for them. Give a few of them a call and see how you are treated and whether you think they will be a good fit. Remember, it is about your comfort too.

Now, make a choice. A hospice representative will come out to your home and sign your loved one up, getting you started.

Hospice A

I liked this about them.... ______________________________

____

____

____

I didn't like this about them.... ________________________

____

____

____

Hospice B

I liked this about them.... ______________________________

____

____

____

I didn't like this about them.... ____________________

Hospice C

I liked this about them.... ____________________

I didn't like this about them.... ____________________

Hospice I chose: ____________________

ELIGIBILITY FOR HOSPICE

Find out if your loved one

- is on or eligible for Medicare (you need their ID number)

- has insurance that covers Hospice (find contact info for the company as well as member id)

- has other financial resources (what are they?)

Now, call the Hospice you have decided upon and give them the information and let them get started getting your loved one enrolled and receiving care.

JOURNAL

As I partner with Hospice...

Chapter Three

FIRST EMOTIONS AS YOU SET OUT

How did it get so late so soon?
It's night before it's afternoon.
December is here before it's June.
My goodness how the time has flewn.
How did it get so late so soon?

~Dr. Seuss

This is it. You are setting out. Your loved one is enrolled in hospice, the family has talked, decisions have been made, a course has been set, and you are about to move away from the shoreline you have always known.

Be warned, the beginning of this journey is filled with strong emotions.

WHAT YOUR LOVED ONE MIGHT BE FEELING

Denial: They might still insist they can do what is no longer possible. They may plan for events that they know they will never be able to attend. They may insist that they don't need help with daily tasks. Don't argue with them. Let them process this. It is part of the grief. They will eventually come to acceptance.

They do know they are dying, but we all want to live. They are coping with the news in bite-size pieces. It will take some time for them to accept the news in both their mind and their heart. As they do, they will allow more help and settle in for the journey.

Loneliness: Dying, by definition, is something one does alone—much like birth. They may be going through this alone, but they do not have to feel lonely. You cannot understand what they are feeling and thinking, but don't pull away from them. You are needed, and your presence brings comfort.

Anger: They might express anger. They are grieving, and anger can be a part of *grief*. Their anger might come your way but probably isn't about you. In fact, it might be coming from *fear*. Anger makes a fearful person feel more in control. It makes them feel that they have some power when they feel so very *powerless* over the situation. "The words of those in pain are like the wind," let them blow by you.

Anger can also come because of *physical pain*. Ask if they are in pain. If so, have your hospice come up with a plan to help manage this.

Fear: There are many unknowns coming for them. They are wondering what this journey will be like. Will it hurt? Will it be embarrassing? Will my wishes be ignored? What comes after death? Assure them that you will treat them with dignity, not leave them and walk with them through this whole journey. If they wish, pray with them and ask God to give them strength and His presence.

Grief: Even though they are still here, they are already thinking of the losses to come. Family, friends, work, hobbies, everything is about to end for them. They are losing who they were in the roles they played. They are losing what they had and those they love. Grief hurts on many levels.

Moving toward death is a letting-go of life. That, unfortunately, brings the feeling of great loss. They need to process through this. You can be there to love them through it.

Victimization: As their ability to make decisions is removed, they can feel out of control and like a victim of their circumstances. This may affect their ability to deal with their illness and can bring a sense of hopelessness.

Educate them as much as they want on their illness. Go to the library, search on the Internet and find out what they want to know. Find answers to their questions or help them obtain them. When they understand what is happening to them, they will feel less at the mercy of the process and more in control of the care they receive.

Encourage them to talk with you about the kind of care they want and don't want. Let them keep control in as many ways as possible as long as possible. This is their life, after all.

Questioning: Your loved one may suddenly seem to have changed their mind. They may tell you something that seems the complete opposite of what they have said before. They are taking inventory of their life and beliefs. This is normal. They are searching for meaning and this is a common part of the process. Listen and help them talk this through if they want. Don't panic as they question. It will help them come to the answers they seek. Be with them in the questions.

WHAT YOU MIGHT BE FEELING

Denial: It is hard to accept what is happening and your mind is probably full of questions and arguments. You may not be able to grasp what is being asked of you as their caregiver. These ups and downs are part of the grief process. Know that it will change and settle down.

Anger: Why them? Why now? Why me? Anger occurs when things feel out of control and unexpected. Anger happens when we are helpless to do anything about it. The best way to deal with anger is to write letters that you never intend to send and then destroy them. You can write to the disease, your loved one, yourself, God. Getting the anger up and out of you will help reduce it. Also, writing out your emotions will help you process them. As you write, you will start to make sense of what you are feeling and put it into perspective. You may even find some solutions.

Fear: What do I say to them? What if I can't do this? There is the unknown, the unexpected, and death itself coming. You probably feel unprepared and ill-equipped for this journey. This book is one way to quell your fear. Becoming educated and equipped will take away much of the uncertainty. As you know what to do and what to expect the unknown will become a smaller and smaller part of what can cause you fear.

Hurt: You don't want to lose your loved one, and it hurts to think of watching them die. You may already be feeling the loss. I know it hurts. I know this is hard. But they are still here and there is time left to spend loving them.

Grief: There is much you are about to lose. You are losing your loved one and their interaction in your life. Holidays will come and go without them. You will want to call, but your loved one will not be here. What should be and could be are about to disappear.

As you start caring for them on this journey, you will lose the normality of your daily life. In the same way that a new birth in the home changes daily life, so does the journey to the end of life—though it is a period of time with an ending. For now, it will be a huge upheaval, but it will be rewarding and transformative. You may look back on this time, thankful for it.

Grief starts with the diagnosis and continues on past the funeral. It will come in stages and with every downturn in your loved one's condition. This grieving can be a time of great growth and I will help you to move through this well.

Love: Amazingly, this journey can deepen and grow your love to levels you never knew. This time can make you more vulnerable, drop your walls, and make you ready and able to love and be loved

Unbalanced and out of control: You may feel at the mercy of all that is happening and feel inadequate to deal with it. This is certainly out of your comfort zone in so many ways. But, here again, is potential for great personal growth. Being out of our comfort zone teaches us new ways to cope and helps to stretch us beyond ourselves.

HOW TO HELP THEM

Treat them the same. They are not their disease or their experiences. Continue treating them as mom or friend or whatever role they played in your life. They are still a whole person with needs on many levels.

You can listen. They still have things to tell you. There are stories to be spoken, and they can still teach, learn, and experience life. Don't focus on the body that is dying but on the spirit that still lives in them.

Let them talk. They do need, and probably want, to talk about this journey and process it. Your job is to be there when they are ready. Just listen. Let them talk and share from their heart whatever they feel. Their emotions might swing wildly at first or they may seem to be emotionless. This is the beginning of the journey, and they will respond uniquely to it. Encourage them to tell you how they feel.

Honor their style of communication. It may be very different than yours and probably won't change now that they are ill. Be mindful of gender, social, and other differences in these difficult times.

They may not want to talk with you but with someone else who feels safe. Don't take that personally. Perhaps there is a support group, a counselor, or close friend with whom they would feel more comfortable talking. Remember, what is most important is helping them find what they need.

Honor their silence. When they need to be quiet and introspective, honor that. They may want to speak with some people and cut off communication with others. They don't have to talk, but you should be ready to listen.

Protect their limits. Help them to not overextend themselves physically, emotionally, or mentally. Help them listen to what their body is telling them and to plan their life today around these limits.

HOW TO HELP YOURSELF

Be **patient with yourself**. And don't be hard on yourself. If you were to think of a friend being in this situation, I'm sure you would be able to give them more grace and understanding than you probably do yourself.

Support group. Find a support group of friends and family or an actual support group. You need help and encouragement right now.

Pray. A lot. God is with you even if you don't feel Him. He is listening. You might as well talk with Him.

Have fun. It is okay to still enjoy life. Your range might be limited as you find you stay home most of the time with your loved one, but you can still be creative. Laughter is a very good medicine and just renting a comedy might lift everyone's spirits.

Journal. My journaling lead to this book. I kept it open on my computer. It was a place to chronicle my journey. In fact, you can read it at the back of this book. When I go back and reread it now, there is so much I had already forgotten. This record of your journey will be valued in the years to come.

Take your vitamins. I know, that sounds like your Mom, but it is important. This is a very stressful time, and you need to ensure that you keep up your strength. Fail to do this, and there is a good chance you will be getting weak and/or sick just when you need your strength.

Have others pray for you. Just knowing that others are lifting you up and thinking about you is a wonderful feeling.

As you set out and you see the land behind you disappear, there will likely be very strong emotions. They are okay to have. But there is also much to do. So, let's look at the details that will help ensure a successful and peaceful passage.

CHAPTER THREE WORKBOOK

What my loved one is expressing... ______________________________

____

____

____

____

Their support group and resources... ______________________________

____

____

____

____

What I am feeling... ______________________________

____

____

____

____

My support group and resources... ______________________________

____

____

____

____

How I will care for myself... ______________________________

____

____

____

____

JOURNAL

I am angry about... ____

I am afraid of... ____

I am losing... ____

What I love... ____

Chapter Four

TAKING INVENTORY AND COUNTING THE COSTS

I try to take one day at a time, but sometimes several days attack me at once.
~Jennifer Yane

YOU ARE HERE

X marks the spot. You are about to embark on a journey, but before you do—let's look at where you are and how you will get to your journey's end.

YOU WILL BE THE CAPTAIN OF THE SHIP

As the main caregiver, you will be leading this journey. It will be up to you to keep it on course and steer clear of dangerous waters. So, we start with you.

You may be willing to volunteer for much more than you can actually do. Think through your time, resources, and support for this journey. By really focusing on this now you can set up a system to effectively manage this passage. Diving in without planning might just do great harm.

A dying person can become as helpless and dependent as a new infant. That means bathing, dressing, feeding, and even diapers.

In addition, you may have to become a nurse, therapist, organizer, spiritual advisor, companion, and confidant. Much of this you will learn as you go. Hands-on experience often teaches us more than any other way.

Hospice will provide you with expert advice, assistance, and intermittent care. However, most of the day-to-day caregiving will be up to you.

You will need to be aware of your own need for care in order to have the resources to care for your loved one. Taking care of yourself makes everything else you do possible.

That means you need to care for yourself physically, planning against burnout and exhaustion. You need to care for yourself mentally by having someone to talk with as you go through this stressful time. Emotionally, you need to give yourself permission to not be tough when you need to cry or stoic when you need to laugh. And, spiritually, you must surround yourself with those who will pray for and with you. Don't forget to spend some time alone with God.

There will be much to do, and, yes, you can delegate. Delegating doesn't make you unable; it just means that you are human and may need help accomplishing the many things that you have to do. It is not a sign of weakness, but strength, to ask for help. Yes, I'm sure you CAN do it all – for a while. Eventually, this pace will catch up with you, and you will find yourself sick or burned out—or both.

In addition, allowing others to help is a blessing to them at a time when there is little they can do. It helps to bring them on the journey, too. They will look back on this time as one in which they were able to care for the loved one even if it was just doing an errand.

CAN YOU HIRE HELP?

This could enable you to spend more time with your family, work part time, have respite or just have additional hands.

You could hire someone to help with the housework, errands or with caregiving. It could be a few hours a day or a few days a week. Extra help can give you a bit more breathing room and, they may even do some things better than you can.

If you hire someone yourself, you will have to pay taxes and/or social security. If you hire from an agency, they will do this for you but these services are generally more expensive.

EXAMINE YOUR CURRENT STAGE OF LIFE

Unless you live alone, this process will impact those who live with you. Likewise, unless you are independently wealthy this will impact your finances and career. Finally, unless you never sleep, this will impact your health, rest, and energy.

Many caregivers will also be married and raising children. Now, you will also be caring for a loved one who is dying.

MARRIAGE IN THE MIDST OF THE JOURNEY

Unfortunately, a dying loved one coming into a home where the marriage is stressed or unhappy will not make it better. Instead, it often exacerbates the issues. But, sometimes, it can cause the couple to draw closer.

It will be essential that you talk about what this journey will look like, the requirements that will be placed on you, and how you will take care of the marriage in the midst of it. Communication is key.

For me, every evening after we got Mom settled in bed, my husband and I would sit outside together. Sometimes we would talk a lot. Others we would just be quiet. Taking that little bit of time each night kept us current in our relationship.

During our evenings together my husband asked me twice whether I wanted to transfer Mom into a full-time care facility. He saw me getting little sleep and the load getting heavier. I was working part-time and he helped me as much as he could, but care-giving was mostly on me. I listened to his concerns, but I really desired to care for my Mom until she died. Nonetheless, talking this through helped us to decide to ask for help. We asked our daughter and her husband to come for two weeks in order to give me some help and some rest.

We worked together through this time, and we grew even closer while caring for my loved one.

IT'S TOUGH TO HAVE A CAREER RIGHT NOW

At first, I was able to work part-time from my home. Mom was ambulatory and didn't need constant help. But as time passed and she needed more assistance and attention, I was no longer able to work.

My sister and I agreed that I would pay myself for caring for Mom out of her accounts. I did not feel great about this, but it enabled me to keep Mom home and pay our bills. I only replaced my income. Hiring help would have been nice so that I could continue working, but it would have cost even more. That was not financially possible.

You may not have the same options as I did. Having to quit or take leave of a job temporarily will mean a loss of income. It could also interfere with your career path. I guess this is the time to decide what is best for you, your family and future, and for your loved one. Check with your company to see if they have leave available for a dying loved one. If not, see if you can take an unpaid leave for a set amount of time. I know this is a tough decision to make. There is wisdom in many counselors so seek good advice here.

LET'S TALK ABOUT THE CHILDREN

Your children will be going through this, too. However, they don't have the resources to understand this, handle it well, and care for themselves in this situation. They will need your help too.

Tell them as much truth, and not more, that they can understand at their age and maturity level. Answer their questions simply, honestly, and, again, according to how much they want to know and how much they can understand.

Reassure them that they are loved. Let them know that they will be cared for. A lot of time and attention will go toward your loved one and less to them. Reassurance is absolutely essential right now. Let them know that just because you have to spend more time with your loved one now does not mean that it will always be this way.

Understand that they may become jealous of the time and attention the loved one is getting. Involve them to the degree they can and to the degree they want to. They can certainly sit in the room and color while you are serving your loved one dinner, for example.

Let them know that it is okay for them to still be a child. There is nothing wrong with them wanting to play, see their friends and act their age. Don't force them to suddenly mature into adulthood because of the stress and seriousness of what you are experiencing.

Reassure them that life will go on. Just because a loved one is dying does not mean that they will suddenly become ill and die. Funny things happen in the mind of a child, so don't assume that they understand what you understand.

Help them to process in an age appropriate way. They can draw what they feel, for example. They may become suddenly clingy, almost as if they have regressed. Just know that this is how they are dealing with the stress. Hug and love them, reassure them, and they will become less needy.

Don't try to protect them from death, you can't. They do know about death. Leaves die, pets die, and death is always on television. Death is part of life for all of us.

We don't want to cause them to focus on death, we want to make sure that they don't come up with their own conclusions about it.

- If you use the term "go to sleep" for death then they might fear bedtime.
- If you don't teach them that not every illness causes death, then they might be afraid of even simple illnesses like the common cold.
- If you say "God will take your loved one home," then they might become afraid of God and that He will take you away from them.
- If you show them that death is a horrible and frightening thing rather than a part of every life and a transition to life with God, then they will have a fear of death that crosses over into all parts of their lives.

Your children are watching you. They will learn from you how to grieve. If you don't allow yourself to show emotions, then they will come to believe that they must keep their feelings, fears, and hurts to themselves, too. When they see that you are sad sometimes and other times not too sad, then they learn that it is okay to feel and that emotions change. Let them know that their feelings are okay and valid.

Show them that your loved one is not dead, but alive. He or she is still the same person that you love.

Help them to grieve. Listen for opportunities to talk with them. Listen for fears and hurts. Let them talk without trying to fix it. Grieving people, and children, need to talk. Be there with them. Answer questions when they come up. Love them always.

Teach them that the dying of a loved one hurts our hearts. For a while we won't be able to see them or talk with them. They will be greatly missed, but there is a reunion coming later. **Give hope**.

BE WILLING TO CHANGE EVERYTHING

It is said that at the end of life we won't regret not working more. We won't regret not having enough hobbies or wealth or stuff. But we will regret the relationships that we did not do well. We will regret not loving enough, caring enough. We will regret that we took those around us for granted.

At the end of our lives, we will look back at people, including ourselves, and see that this is what life was about. Right now, you may have to undergo significant changes in your daily life, but you are investing in the people in your life and that will pay you dividends forever.

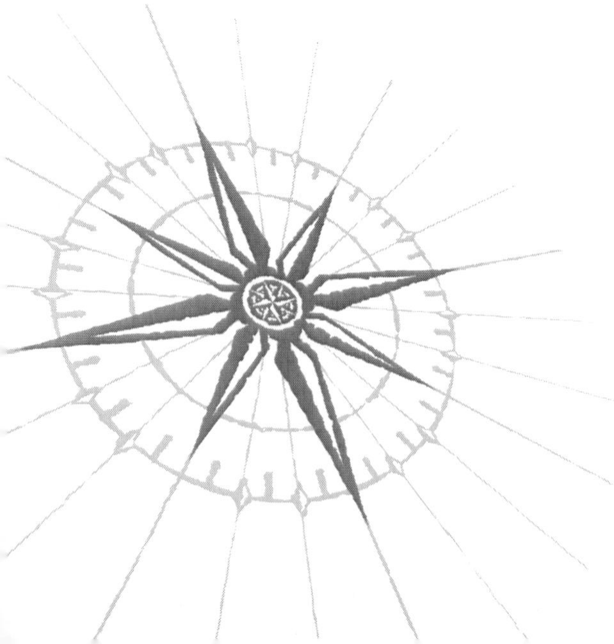

CHAPTER FOUR WORKBOOK

List all your roles and the time you spend at each.

Now, what can you delegate, move, delete, or revise in order to have the time and resources to devote to caring for your loved one and yourself? Know your limitations.

How will you care for your relationships?

Spouse – ____

____

____

____

____

____

Family – ____

____

____

____

____

____

Friends – ____

____

____

____

____

____

Career – ____

____

____

____

____

____

JOURNAL

As I look at the roles I play in life... ____________________

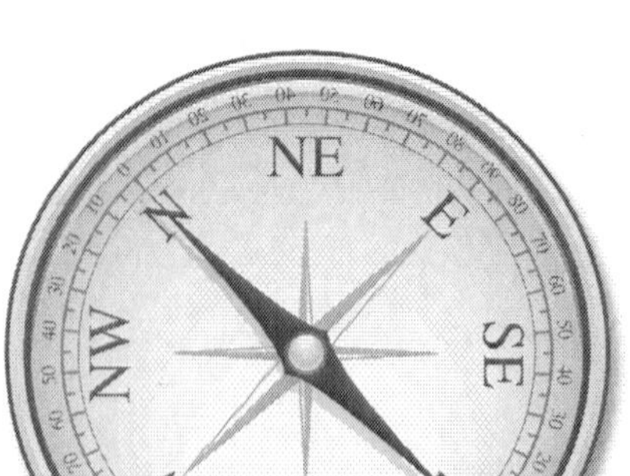
N
NE
E
SE
S
SW
W
NW

Chapter Five

SETTING SAIL

Every one of us has in him a continent of undiscovered character. Blessed is he who acts the Columbus to his own soul.

~Author Unknown

There are going to be joys and pitfalls on this journey…and lack of sleep, stress, and a few laughs as well. Your goal is to do your best, and that is all you can do. You just need a bit of help getting started.

ORGANIZE THE CAREGIVERS

This experience is about comfort and alleviating discomfort under constantly changing circumstances. Making a schedule will be a huge help in accomplishing this.

Being organized and scheduled will bring back some control to a situation that feels completely out of your control. You can even schedule time for yourself and your family.

Get input – those who are going to be directly involved in the caring should get to be part of developing the plan. If they are part of the planning, they are more likely to stay involved in the execution of the plan. So, ask for input on the organizing and caregiving.

Rather than dictating, ask how each person feels they can best help. Allow them to serve in the way that is most like them. Others would prefer to be directed so be ready to do this as well. In both cases, be clear about what is expected as well as the limitations.

ORGANIZE THE CAREGIVING

Now, we need to talk about the equipment you will need for this journey. Getting this together now will help later. Make sure you enlist the caregivers too.

Set up the bedroom: Before my mother moved in with us, I repainted the room and bought new curtains. I had asked her what she wanted from her home so we could put out pictures and knickknacks. I wanted the room to feel like home for her.

I organized all the things we will talk about below, and when Mom came I felt prepared. Well, at least as much as I could be. Here are some areas to think through ahead of time.

Separate the trash and laundry: It is best to have a large, covered trash with liners in your loved one's bedroom. As you use medical supplies, tissues, and other disposables, they should be separated from the rest of the family. Buy a large box of trash bags. You will go through quite a few over the days.

A separate laundry hamper is absolutely essential. You will go through a lot of linens, and some might be soiled. It is best not to mix this laundry with the family laundry. This also ensures that you will be able to have their needs attended to quickly.

Prepare linens: Later in the book, you will see how to layer a bed so that you can remove soiled linens and have another set underneath ready to go. You will also be using flat sheets as draw sheets to help you move them in bed. This means you will need extra linens. Keeping these extra linens in your loved one's room will mean one less step for you.

Organize and gather dishes: In the beginning, you will use normal dishes. However, you may need to improvise so that your loved one can manage eating and drinking as time passes. Consider lidded sippy cups, straws, a serving tray, etc.

Retrofit the bathroom: Buy a tub chair, bath mats, and a grab bar. Ask Hospice to deliver an elevated toilet seat. You will likely need an in-room potty over the coming days. I didn't want one, but when Mom could no longer walk a potty by her bed turned out to be a godsend. Hospice will provide an inflatable tub for washing hair while lying down in bed as well as a no-rinse shampoo.

Buy or separate out towels to be used only by your loved one. These will probably need to be laundered separately.

Get a hospital bed: While your loved one might not like the idea of being in a hospital bed now, being able to raise and lower the bed and head and feet will be a blessing for you later. This is covered by hospice under medical equipment. Hospice can generally deliver a bed within a day.

SAFETY FIRST

- Put away throw rugs or put down nonskid backing.
- Use a cane, walker, and wheelchair as needed (hospice will provide these).
- Put stickers on sliding glass doors.
- Make the transitions between different types of flooring as even as you can.
- Check the handrails on stairwells and make sure there are nonskid treads on wooden stairs.
- Arrange furniture to make pathways accessible.
- Pad the sharp edges on tables and chairs.
- Keep medications away from children.
- Add lighting to ensure safety at night.
- Use monitors to hear or view your loved when you are not in the room.

ORGANIZING THE DETAILS

Have a place for everything and everything in its place. Keeping what you need in one place shortens the time spent finding items in different rooms and keeps them all where you will use them. For example:

- Place a cart, large basket, or tub that contains the immediate supplies you need in your loved one's room (bathing, sanitary, etc.).
- Keep all towels and linens to be used by your loved one in his/her room, if possible—or all together in another area.
- Keep a pad of paper to list questions for hospice, so that you will not forget when they are visiting.
- Keep all medications in one place (and away from the kids).
    - Use a one-week, multi-time dispenser and fill it once per week. This alerts you to needed refills ahead of time and you can see at-a-glance if you have dispensed the needed medications.
- Have a phone list posted by the phone.
    - Sort the list by type: doctor, hospice, pharmacy; family and friends; people who can help with errands, etc.
- Create a phone tree to keep everyone updated and for when you need extra help.
    - You call one person who agrees to call one or two others who agree to pass on the information.
- Keep a list of who agreed to help with:
    - general errands
    - laundry
    - housekeeping
    - transportation
    - nighttime care

  - caring for visiting friends and family
  - emergency help
  - shopping
  - pet care
  - legal issues
  - funeral planning
  - returning phone calls
  - updating the web site
  - getting medical supplies and equipment not provided by hospice
- Train your helpers.
  - Determine the kind of help you need, how much help you need, and for how long.
  - Spend time up front showing what kind of help you need and how you need it. This will make it easier to let go and focus on your loved one.

VISITORS

Ask your loved one who s/he would like to visit, and only allow those people to come. No one has the right to see your loved one at this time without permission.

Don't let visitors drain you or your loved one. Set boundaries on when visits can occur and for how long. Arrange visits at your convenience, not the visitors'. They are coming to minister to your loved one, not be waited upon. Keep a list handy of how they can help, and allow them to care for you and your loved one through serving you.

KEEP EVERYONE INFORMED

Use www.caringbridge.org to keep everyone up to date. Caring Bridge is a nonprofit organization dedicated to helping families who are going through major illnesses and are a huge blessing. Caringbridge.org is a free service that provides a private web site for you and your loved one. It helps to keep everyone in the loop. It ends the constant phone calls and having to repeat the same things many times. I heard of this after my mother had passed and wished I had learned of it sooner.

The web site allows you to update information as needed. It also allows friends and family to comment. People can also upload pictures and the comments and pictures can be compiled into an album later for a minimal cost.

PLAN AHEAD

Surround yourself with those who will encourage, support, and affirm you. Find those who will pray for you and with you. Get your support system in place now.

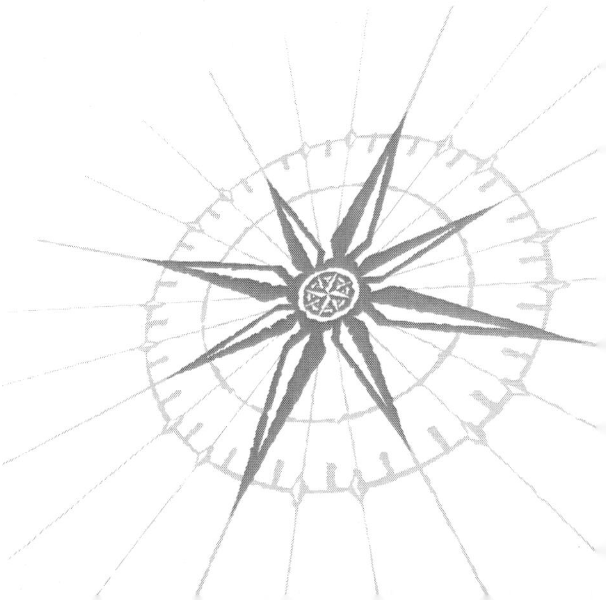

CHAPTER FIVE WORKBOOK

List the caregivers and their jobs. ______________________________

Make a phone list of everyone you need or will call on.

What do you need to organize the

- Bedroom ______________________________

____

____

____

____

- Linens ______________________________

____

____

____

____

- Dishes ______________________________

____

____

____

____

- Bathroom ______________________________

____

____

____

____

- Medical equipment ______________________________

____

____

____

____

____

____

Safety needs ______________________________

____

____

____

____

____

____

Medications list ______________________________

____

____

____

____

____

____

Visitor hours or guidelines ______________________________

____

____

____

____

____

____

Who will set up and update caringbridge.org? ______________________________

____

____

____

____

JOURNAL

Write about what you are doing well each day. Encourage yourself.

Write about your regrets and what you can do about them. Do what you can and throw the rest overboard.

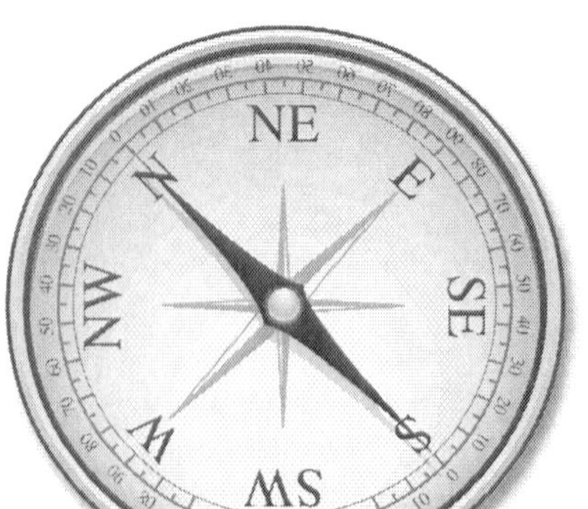
NE
E
SE
S
SW
W
NW
N

Chapter Six

HANDS ON DECK: THE BASICS OF CARING

For a long time it had seemed to me that life was about to begin—real life. But there was always some obstacle in the way. Something to be got through first, some unfinished business, time still to be served, a debt to be paid. Then life would begin. At last it dawned on me that these obstacles were my life.

~Fr. Alfred D'Souza

KEEP A CHART

On it you will notate whatever you need to keep track of or let hospice know.

- This chart can be as detailed as you want, listing food, bowel, meds, etc.
- This chart can be a list of questions or concerns so you won't forget.

EATING AND DRINKING

"Chocolate, chocolate, chocolate" was my Mom's wish for food. She would be happy with it at every meal. Normally, we wouldn't give this "food" so often to a loved one, but it helped her to eat. She wanted it and, what the heck, it made her happy. At this stage, it is important for your loved one to be eating, period. If there are foods that s/he is craving, it is best to indulge. Mom would eat other things as well, but chocolate was a sweet treat that she enjoyed, and enjoyed daily.

We are very concerned with getting our loved one to eat but this may become difficult for them. You can try smaller more frequent meals: think of snacking or grazing instead of full, heavy meals. It is important to keep the calorie intake constant as long as possible.

Ask what your loved one wants to eat. When you are ill, certain things seem repulsive and some things sound very good to eat. Get a feel for what sounds appealing and prepare this type of meal.

Try to keep your loved one hydrated. Dehydration can cause complications. As your loved one is less mobile s/he will require less liquid, but will tend to drink even less than this.

You can try popsicles as a way to bring in more fluids. When your loved one stops drinking, you can swab their mouth and use lip balm to keep their lips from chapping.

See what doesn't work and make changes.

Keep the following in mind.

- Medications may affect appetite.

- Mouth and throat sores make it harder to eat and swallow.
- Avoid high fat as they are harder to digest.
- Try blander and familiar foods.
- Stick to familiar and favorite foods.
- Crackers can help with nausea.

As it becomes difficult to eat

- Make foods thicker as this is easier to swallow. The following may be preferable:
    - casseroles
    - hot cereals
    - canned fruits
    - egg dishes like quiche
    - well cooked vegetables in sauce
    - egg, tuna, or meat salads
    - cottage or cream cheese
    - puddings and custards
    - juices and smoothies with added nutrients
    - gelatin and ice cream
    - milkshakes, yogurt, and eggnog
    - popsicles for extra hydration
- Foods that are difficult to eat.
    - white bread (It is sticky and hard to swallow.)
    - mashed potatoes served plain
    - peas, corn, rice (They fall off the fork.)
    - banana and peanut butter (They are too thick.)
- Use non-spill cups and flexible straws.

Mealtime.

- Never feed someone lying down as they could choke.
- Make sure they are swallowing well. Have them slow down if necessary.

- Watch for food being "pocketed" in the cheek rather than swallowed.
- It is important to consider infection control. You don't want to bring or spread one.
    - Wash your hands before care.
    - Wear gloves.
    - Disinfect when and where necessary as soon as possible.
    - Use separate trash and plastic bags for loved one's refuse.
    - Keep soiled linens in a plastic bag until laundered. Launder quickly.
    - There will be lots of laundry if mealtime is taking place in bed.
    - Wash your hands at end of care.

BATHING AND HYGIENE

Hospice will provide a CNA to help with bathing and personal hygiene. If possible, I recommend that you let hospice do this for you. This is especially true if your loved one needs help getting in and out of the shower or tub. The CNAs are trained in keeping this very safe. They are skilled in caring for your loved one and will do so with the utmost respect and attention.

If you are going to help with bathing yourself, here are some suggestions:

- Get everything ready ahead of time.
    - basin, water, washcloths, towels, soaps, etc.
    - new clothing for after bath.

- Use a shower seat or lift chair in the tub for safety.
    - Take great care transferring your loved one to the tub (see "Transfers" later in this chapter).
- Wash one part at time. Keep the rest of the body covered when bathing in bed to keep them warm.
- Use no rinse products when bathing in bed.
- Wash hair in bed.
    - Remove the pillow and place the towel and/or waterproof pad under the head to protect the bed.
    - Place the drain from the collection device into bucket on floor.
    - Place the water collection device under loved one's head.
    - Wet hair from pitcher of warm water.
    - Shampoo with no rinse solution.
    - Drain all water into the bucket.
    - Remove device and towel; dry and comb.
- Clean teeth and dentures.
- Shave.

BOWEL AND BLADDER

Although bowel and bladder functions will slow down as the journey progresses, this will still be a daily concern. The first rule is keep your loved one clean and dry to prevent skin sores. Urine and feces can quickly damage the skin and cause sores if not cleaned properly.

Your loved one may be able to use the restroom alone at first. Over time, though, you may need to help him/her to the toilet and offer assistance in being seated. Let your loved one act independently as long as possible. You will most likely be helping more and more in this area as time progresses.

The next stage might be starting to help with cleaning after using the facilities. Then might come an in-room potty when walking to the toilet is too difficult. If your loved one becomes completely bed-bound, then you will be using a urinal and/or bed pan and maybe even diapers.

Here are some tips for this area of care.

- **Always use gloves**!
- Keep your loved one warm while using facilities.
  - If your loved one is on opioid painkillers, employ a stool softener or laxative to prevent constipation.
  - Lack of exercise slows the bowels, too.
- Provide a **raised toilet seat** with bars to assist in getting on and off the toilet. Ask hospice to provide one for you.
- An **in-room potty** can be supplied by hospice when your loved one can't walk to bathroom.
  - How to use the in-room potty.
    - Take care in transferring a loved one onto the seat.
    - Have chux or other waterproof pad under the seat on the floor just in case there is a spill.
    - Pour white vinegar (a cup or two) into the bucket and keep lid on when not in use. The vinegar absorbs the smell and the lid on the bucket keeps the vinegar smell out of the room. We kept a gallon container of vinegar in the bathroom.

        - Remove the lid to bucket and help loved one onto the seat.
        - When your loved one is finished, make sure s/he is clean and transfer him/her back to bed or chair.
        - Place the lid on bucket and take it to the bathroom.
    - How to clean the in-room potty.
        - Pour urine and/or feces into the toilet then rinse the bucket with water and pour that into the toilet. Put in more vinegar, replace the lid, and put the bucket back into the potty in the bedroom.

- **Bed pan and Urinal** (When your loved one can no longer get out of bed.)
    - How to use the urinal.
        - Place the urinal between the legs.
        - Assist your loved one in placing the penis into the urinal, if necessary.
        - Hold the urinal, if needed.
        - Allow your loved one to wipe.
        - Provide hand-washing materials.
    - How to use a bed pan.
        - Have your loved one bend knees and raise hips.
        - Slide the bedpan into place under your loved one.
        - Raise the head of the bed or use pillows to help them into a more upright position.
        - Allow your loved one to wipe or assist with this.

        - Lower the head of the bed or remove pillows and then remove bedpan.
        - Help your loved one to clean hands.
    - How to clean urinal and bed pan.
        - Empty contents into the toilet.
        - Rinse and empty again into toilet.
        - You can swish with vinegar and then discard this into the toilet and rinse one more time, if necessary.

- **Diapers** are used when your loved one becomes incontinent either intermittently or continually. Hospice will supply these for you; there are many different types. We tried several until we found a brand that worked well for my mother. Unfortunately, diapers can raise the chances of certain skin problems. Here are some tips:
    - Use a Chux pad under your loved one in bed in case there is a leak; hospice will supply you with these.
    - With your loved one on his/her back, undo the diaper tabs and pull the front down between the legs folding it in on itself to keep the wet part inside.
    - Clean your loved one well. Always clean from front to back.
    - Fold one side of the diaper and tuck it under your loved one's hip.
    - Roll your loved one onto the folded side and pull the diaper out from under the hip, removing.
    - Clean the anal area well.
    - Roll the old Chux pad with the wet part to the inside and tuck that under the hip your loved one is currently lying on.

- Partially roll a new Chux and push that under the old one under the hip while keeping the rest of the Chux flat. (Your loved one will be rolling back onto the flat part.)
- Place a new diaper on your loved while s/he is still on his/her side tucking part under their hip. (The new Chux will already be in place.)
- Roll your loved one onto his/her back, rolling your loved one onto the new diaper and new Chux.
- Roll gently toward you to pull the old Chux from under your loved one's hip and the tucked part of new diaper to the front.
- Bring the diaper up between the legs.
- Attach tabs.

- **Changing the bed with your loved one in it.** If you start with your loved one out of the bed you can put down several layers of bedding at once. You can do this with them in the bed but you would have to roll them a few times as you will see.
  - Put on a flat sheet.
  - Place another flat sheet folded into thirds across the middle of the bed where your loved one's torso will be. This is called a "draw sheet" and you can tuck the overhang under the mattress.
  - Place a chux on top of that.
  - Put a rubber sheet or pad over this.
  - Repeat this process again.
  - Repeat this process again – you now have three layers of bedding. Place a top sheet and blanket on.
  - Your loved one will lie on top of these three layers.

As one becomes soiled roll your loved one onto their side, undo the flat sheet from the top and bottom, roll it like a tootsie roll toward their back and tuck it under the hip they are lying on. Roll them onto the clean flat sheet underneath and remove the rest of the rolled soiled sheet. You can do this two more times before you reach the exposed mattress.

- Replace the cover sheet and blanket if needed.

SKIN HYGIENE AND PROBLEMS

Once a skin sore starts, it is a lot of work to not only get rid of it but to keep it from getting worse. The immune system may not be functioning well as your loved one gets sicker and so a skin sore is even more difficult to treat. **Prevention is your first goal.**

Skin sores can start because of constant pressure on a particular area. You can work against this by:

- changing your loved one's position every 2 to 3 hours
- using pillows to prop him/her up and remove any pressure
- placing an egg-crate foam pad under your loved one

Skin sores can also start from being wet. Ensuring that your loved one is clean and dry will take extra commitment, especially as s/he becomes bedridden or use diapers. Prevention is actually easier than treatment.

- Always ensure your loved one is completely dry before dressing or placing a new diaper.
- Change diapers as often as you need to, not on set intervals.
- Cover vulnerable areas with a protective water repellent.

Stages of skin breakdown

- Stage 1: Damage can be reversed by relieving pressure.
    - Skin is red but intact, lasting 15-30 minutes.
    - Redness and heat are at a particular pressure point.
    - Treatment
        - Change positions often.
        - Don't massage the area, as it is already sensitive.
        - Use a pillow or sheepskin or flotation pad to take the pressure off the area.
- Stage 2
    - There is a partial breakdown of skin thickness.
    - Appears as an abrasion or scrape or a blister.
    - Treatment
        - Call hospice for advice on treatment.
        - Wound needs to be cleaned; hospice will advise on salves or dressings needed.
- Stage 3
    - There is a full breakdown in skin thickness.
    - All layers of the skin are destroyed.
    - There may be a thick, scab-like material.
    - Treatment
        - Follow the same instructions as in stage 2 but realize that you are dealing with a more serious skin breakdown so be extra careful with cleaning and care.
- Stage 4
    - Skin loss, with extensive damage.
    - Skin is dead and there may be damage to the muscle, supporting structures, or bone.

- Treatment
    - Hospice will advise.
    - May require temporary in-patient treatment.

Once a skin breakdown occurs, at best it will be an ongoing headache; at worst, it is a nightmare. Do all that you can to prevent skin breakdowns. Should this sort of condition arise, be sure to follow hospice's advice to avoid worsening the condition. Mom had a Stage 2-3 area on her buttocks when she came to live with me. We worked hard to get it healed but were only able to keep it from getting worse no matter what we did. Prevention. Prevention. Prevention.

EXERCISE

Movement of any kind helps circulation, alleviates some stiffness and soreness, and helps with constipation. While for you, exercise may be aerobics, weights, long walks, or runs, for our purposes, exercise is simply movement.

You can help someone who is bed-bound with range of motion exercises. Neck, shoulder, arm, leg, hip, etc. can all be stretched and flexed. It would be a good idea to have hospice send a physical therapist to teach you the best range of motion movements for your loved one.

TRANSFERS

You may need to assist your love one in moving from one place to another. You can hurt yourself and your loved one if you don't do this correctly. I took a big fall when moving my mother from her potty to her bed because I wasn't paying attention to what I was doing. Luckily, she was not hurt, but I hit the dresser and was badly bruised and sore for a week.

Lifting techniques: In order to move your loved one from one place to another, first make sure that the desired location is 45 degrees to the side. Stand in front of your loved one and position yourself for the transfer. Place your knees on either side of his/hers and have your loved one place his/her arms around your neck if they can. Bend your knees and keep your back straight. Place your arms under your loved one's arms and hold the shoulder blades with your palms. Tell your loved one you are going to lift him/her and count to three. Stand up with your loved one. Now, help your loved one to pivot with you to the chair or bed or potty. Lower your loved one into place and make sure s/he is stable and secure.

Moving in bed: People tend to slide down in bed, especially if you have a hospital bed that you place in the raised position. You will need to pull your loved one up from time to time. This is where a **draw sheet** comes in handy.

A **draw sheet** is a flat sheet that has been folded in half or in thirds and lays on top of the fitted sheet on the bed. You can place a waterproof Chux (hospice will supply these for you) over that. Your loved one lies directly on this draw sheet and Chux. When you want to move your loved one up in bed, lower the head of the bed and raise the legs a bit. Have your loved one bend his/her knees. At this point, you should position yourself behind your loved one and looking at his/her head. Grab a good portion of the draw sheet on either side of your loved one in each hand. Have your loved one give a little push with his/her bent legs and pull up on the draw sheet. Since the torso is lying on the draw sheet you will pull your loved one's entire body upward.

The draw sheet is also a great help in repositioning your loved one. In order to move your loved one from his/her back to side reach across them and grab the draw sheet and pull toward you. Your loved one will roll with the sheet. After you have positioned your loved one, you can lay the draw sheet flat again.

Always remember to use good body mechanics. You can pull a muscle or really hurt yourself moving another person. My mother weighed only five pounds less than I did, but I was able to move her from bed to potty or wheelchair and back again by myself when I paid attention and followed these steps.

AMBULATION

Your loved one may need help moving and walking. Initially, s/he may be able to walk. Soon, this might progress to needing help getting up and staying steady with a walker or cane and then to needing a wheelchair. My mother went from needing help walking to being completely unable to walk in a matter of hours. Luckily, hospice delivered a wheelchair almost immediately, or I would not have been able to help her back to bed.

A **transfer belt** might be a big help getting your loved one from a seated to a standing position and even keeping him/her steady with their cane or walker. Hospice will provide this for you and show you how to use it. Personally, I found that just good lifting techniques and paying attention worked for me.

SLEEP

Without sleep you will become unable to function well, let alone care for another who is dependent upon you. Even ensuring six hours a night will be a big help. **Monitors** can be a big help here, too.

Placing a monitor next to your and your loved one's bed means that you will be able to hear if your loved one calls for help or if there is a noise. A video monitor is the best. You can turn off the video and just listen while you are in bed, but if you hear something you can turn on the video to see that your loved one was just changing positions and go back to sleep yourself. These video monitors work in a very dark room, so there is no need to keep on a potentially bothersome light.

Since you need your sleep, you need to ensure your loved one is also getting rest. If your loved one is having trouble sleeping, you can talk to hospice about medications. Hospice will work with you to find the right one and the right dosage so that everyone will get some rest.

MEDICATIONS

A weekly dispenser is best to use if you have more than one or two medications. On a specific day of the week, you place all medications into the appropriate day and time slots for the full week. At a glance, you can see whether you need more medications or see whether you remembered to dispense the medications that morning. Also, keep all of your medications in one place and away from kids and pets. Your hospice nurse will monitor the medications and have them refilled for you.

PAIN MANAGEMENT

The fear of pain and whether or not it can be controlled is a big issue at this point. Since you don't really know what to expect there can be anxiety about this area.

Educate yourself and your loved one on why there is or might be pain, what can be done about it, and what can be done if those methods don't work. Fear amplifies pain, so alleviate fear as best as you can. Give reassurance that everything that can be done to alleviate pain will be done. Give reassurances that s/he will not be alone and in pain. Make sure your loved one knows that it is important to you that s/he be cared for well.

Pain does not always accompany dying. Not every illness causes pain, but it can't always be prevented, either. However, a person shouldn't have to die with a lot of pain, as it can be controlled 90% of the time. If one pain medication isn't working well it can be adjusted, changed, and administered differently as needed.

There are different types of pain. Ask how, how much, where, and when your loved one feels pain. Pain is subjective but always real to the person experiencing it. People also tolerate pain differently. What you want to know about your loved one's pain is whether it is:

- Dull or sharp
- Chronic or acute
- Continual or intermittent
- Unbearable or an annoyance: use a scale from 1-10 to help gauge the level of pain
- In one part of the body or everywhere

Knowing this information will be very helpful when you are working with hospice to find the right medications to treat any pain that might occur.

Pain is physical and emotional. It can expose fears or cause fear. It can be isolating and lonely and even cause a longing for death so it will end. In most cases, the pain can be controlled. Your loved one will need you to stay with him/her and love him/her throughout the experience. Do what you can to alleviate the physical pain while paying close attention to your loved one's emotional reaction to it.

Pain management is the goal. Severe pain causes the loved one to become focused on it and finding relief, rather than on daily life.

- **Stay ahead of the pain.** This means you don't wait until there is a lot of pain to give medication. It is harder to bring pain under control than to simply keep it under control. Ask regularly about the pain your loved one experiences and its level. Administer medication before the pain becomes severe.

- **Find the right medications and dosages.** The medication needs to be right for your loved one, the disease, the pain level, and your loved one's wants. It doesn't have to make your loved one unconscious or incapacitated, but s/he may want to be asleep more rather than experience the pain.

- **Don't worry about addiction.** Addiction is not going to be an issue when we are talking about pain relief. Managing pain is not the same as seeking drugs. Yes, your loved one's dosage may have to increase with time in order to reach the same level of relief, but rest assured, this is not the same as using drugs to get high.

- **Seeing your loved one in pain is very difficult to watch.** It can make you feel helpless and anxious, too. Work closely with hospice if your loved one is in pain until you can find the right combination of therapies to help.

At first, this all may be new to you and a bit overwhelming but you will get the hang of it. Every day you will gain experience and become more comfortable with giving care to your loved one. Don't hesitate to ask your hospice team for help when and where you need it.

WHEN TO CALL HOSPICE FOR HELP

Pain and Swelling

- New or worsening pain
- Your loved one's pain is not regulated by current medication
- Chest pain or tightness
- New or increased pain or redness in swollen area
- New or increased swelling anywhere on the body

Breathing

- It is hard for them to catch their breath
- Inhalers aren't working
- Hard to breathe when lying prone
- Worsening cough
- Change in color, thickness, or odor of spit

Digestion and Urination

- Vomiting
- Nausea
- Vomiting blood
- Persistent diarrhea
- No bowel movements for 3 days
- Pain or difficulty during bowel movement
- Blood in bowel movement
- Leaking colostomy
- Catheter is leaking
- Painful urination
- Blood in urine or cloudy urine
- Stomach feels bloated or swollen
- No urination for one day

Mood

- Constantly feeling anxious
- They are unable to relax
- They are having trouble sleeping

Wounds or Bleeding

- New skin problem
- Change in drainage, amount, color, or odor
- Increased pain or redness at the wound site
- New or increased bleeding from a new or existing wound
- Bleeding that won't stop
- Blood in the catheter or IV
- Blood in the stool, urine, or vomit

Fever and chills

- Temperature is greater than 101
- Can't get warm (chills)
- Sweating or itching

Medication and Equipment

- Need more medications
- Medications are not meeting needs
- Need more information on medications
- Equipment making strange noises or not working
- Need additional equipment or supplies

If in doubt, call your hospice.

CHAPTER SIX WORKBOOK

What I need to organize or where I need help…

- Food and liquids ______________________________

- Bathing and hygiene ______________________________

- Bowel and bladder ______________________________

- Skin issues ______________________________

- Exercise ______________________________

- Pain management ______________________________

- Changes in your loved one on any level ______________________________

- Equipment and/or supplies needed ______________________________

JOURNAL

I am feeling equipped or unequipped and it is causing.... ____

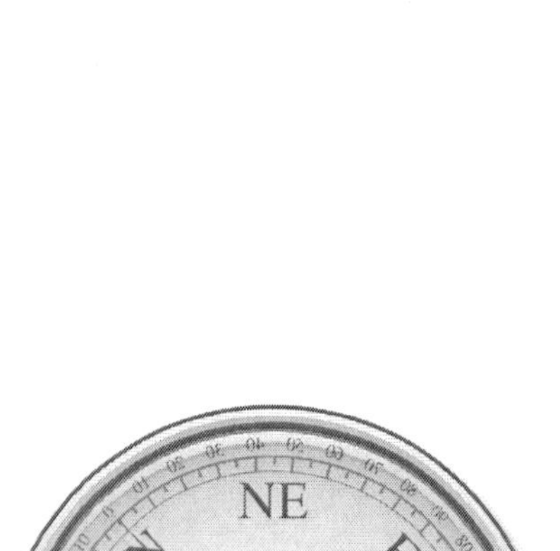
NE
E
SE
S
SW
W
NW
N

Chapter Seven

HERE THERE BE MONSTERS: ENTERING UNCHARTED WATERS

Truth hurts—not the searching after; the running from!

~John Eyberg

Now that you've ventured out on this journey and can no longer see land, things can get a bit scary. You, and your loved one, are truly in uncharted waters. There is no going back.

On very old sailings maps, when the world was not completely explored, inscriptions would warn other sailors of dangerous waters: It would be written on the map, "Here there be monsters." These areas of the ocean were uncharted and thought to be dangerous. These were warnings to keep those who came behind them safe in their passage.

In this chapter, we'll talk about what you and your loved one might be feeling at this stage of the journey and make sure you are not heading toward dangerous waters.

Emotions are changing, heightening, and can be treacherous now. **For your loved one, the most common emotion is fear.** And that fear covers a lot of ground.

FEAR OF LOSING CONTROL

As the body moves closer to death, there will be a loss of control in many areas from bodily functions to communication to movement. Your loved one is moving from independence to dependence and that can be frightening for a person who has cared for him/herself for a very long time. If your loved one has always been very proper, then the thought that he or she may lose dignity is most abhorrent.

How to help: Assure your loved one that you will always protect his/her dignity. Show your loved one from the very beginning by asking about specific wants, opinions, procedures, etc. Reassure your loved one that as s/he does lose some function that you will still provide excellent care.

FEAR OF PAIN AND SUFFERING

Your loved one may not fear death as much as the pain that dying can cause. Knowing that there may be pain and suffering but not knowing for sure or how much or if it can be controlled is again very scary.

How to help: Pain can be an issue, but in over 90% of cases is managed so well that the loved one never really experiences much in the way of suffering. There are so many different medications and therapies that, for the most part, your loved one will not suffer. However, dying can include discomfort. Assure your loved one that you will be very proactive in treating any pain or suffering.

FEAR OF THE UNKNOWN

This fear covers not only what might happen as the disease progresses but also the fear of what happens after death.

How to help: If your loved one can understand, have hospice explain his/her particular disease, what to expect and how they will provide care. Knowledge can help with fear, so provide what you can.

When my mother was dying, she was fearless because she knew where she was going. She experienced anxiety in the process but never feared the outcome.

You can help your loved one by talking with them or having the chaplain talk with them about this after-life. The Bible notes, "what is mortal will be swallowed up by life." Life, not death, awaits us after we leave these mortal bodies.

For those who don't have a spiritual belief, dying can be very frightening. For those who do, after working through unfinished business people often experience peace about what will happen after death. You can help by assisting your loved one to finish life here and making sure that s/he is supported spiritually until then.

FEAR OF UNFINISHED BUSINESS

After a lifetime, there could very well be a lot of unfinished business. This might include unfinished business in relationships, work, finances, spiritual issues, wounds received and given, or old secrets. While this unfinished business may have been buried or ignored before, it will most likely come to the surface now.

How to help: You can ask your loved one if there is someone with whom s/he needs to speak, something they feel they still need to do, etc. If your loved one does share something with you ask how you can help. Maybe you can contact someone and arrange a conversation, for example.

FEAR OF ABANDONMENT AND BEING ALONE

Dying is very much something that one experiences alone, but it is even more frightening to think that you might be abandoned or die with no one by your side. As illness progresses, your loved one may begin to feel left out of the life in the house and a bit lonely.

How to help: If you were to put yourself in your loved one's place, what would you want? Try to understand what it would be like to be on the other side of this journey. Now, with this deeper understanding and compassion, you can care for your loved one and let him/her know that you are committed to being with him/her and will do everything you can to make sure your loved one is not alone.

FEAR OF ACTUALLY DYING

Questions such as, "will it hurt" and "where will I go" do go through the mind of one who is nearing death.

How to help: This area is one that you could refer in part to Hospice. Your RN will have seen many people pass from this life. The RN is the best prepared to speak with your loved one about what s/he knows about the actual death experience.

Your loved one may also experience **depression, anger, grief.** These are all part of processing the life that one has lived and is about to leave behind. It is okay for your loved one to feel these things but take care that s/he doesn't turn into a deep depression or other emotional problems.

How to help: Listen to your loved one. Try to place yourself in your loved one's shoes and see from his/her eyes. Attempt to understand why your loved one acts as s/he does and look for the underlying emotion or need. Your loved one is undergoing a great stress and it will show itself in some ways that are difficult for you. Hang in there with your loved one. This is a process, a journey, and you can be there to love your loved one through it all. And don't forget that Hospice will provide a counselor if needed.

GRIEF

This will be your loved one's constant companion on the journey. Your loved one is slowly losing who s/he was. Friends and family will be gone soon. Your loved one will be looking back on his/her life and seeing regrets, having melancholy emotions, already counting the loss. Life goes on without us when we pass, and there is grief in that thought.

Grief helps us to process, to feel, and to transform. Your loved one needs to experience this. It helps him/her to let go of the past and move forward on this journey.

How to help: Photo albums help your loved one to talk, and people who are grieving need to talk. Let your loved one tell you about his/her life and the people and experiences in that life. Remember, your loved one is reviewing and letting go. Help your loved one.

Let your loved one know that s/he will not be forgotten but cherished and remembered and talked about. Let your loved one know the impact s/he has had on your life and how you are blessed to have known them. Help your loved one to look to the life to come as s/he finishes up the life your loved one had here.

All the emotions we have mentioned can be normal for the journey and you will have to take care to navigate them well so that you can pass through them without being pulled under.

You are also on this journey in these uncharted waters but **your experience will be somewhat different** than your loved one's.

FOR YOU THE EMOTIONS CAN BE A ROLLER COASTER

Your feelings may parallel your loved one's in some ways, but we will talk specifically about your experience here.

STRESS

Stress is a given. You will feel stress. The physical requirements will cause stress as will the emotional, social, spiritual, relational, and mental aspects of your daily life. How you deal with the stress will determine the outcome.

Stress is good for you and bad for you. A bit of stress causes us to sink our roots deep as we are pushed by the winds. Stress is bad for you when it is so intense and continuous that you feel overwhelmed and exhausted.

Consider how to help yourself if the stress is getting to be too much. Set reasonable, obtainable goals and let the rest go.

- Can you break the one big problem into manageable steps?
- Can you deal with each little problem one at a time?
- Can you delegate?
- Can you take a break and breathe and think?
- Do you need outside help?
- Do you need to see your doctor or therapist?

DEPRESSION

Depression comes from anger turned inward and/or blocked goals and frustration. When it takes hold, depression brings about a sense of hopelessness that can cause you to give up and give in.

There is certainly sadness as you care for your dying loved one. Sadness is a normal part of what you are experiencing. Depression is different. It starts with your **self-talk.**

If you really listen to what you are telling yourself, you will find that your emotions follow the flavor of it like a puppy follows you with a toy. If you are telling yourself negative things, then expect your emotions to be down and negative as well. If you make changes in what you tell yourself, you can expect your emotions to change as well.

You can't change what is happening, but you can tell yourself a positive that is true. For example,

> This is sooo difficult (*true*)I feel like I can't take this anymore (*emotions going downhill*), but I can call for help *(a positive that is true*). I can arrange a break tomorrow afternoon. I can remember that God is right here with me and gives me the strength for each moment (*emotions leveling off or coming back up*).

You told yourself the hard truth but ended it with actions that you can take as well as positives that are also true. Listen to what is going on between your ears, and make yourself find the positives to bring back balance.

If your depression is coming from a **blocked goal** and that goal is for your loved one to live but they are dying, then you could experience depression. That blocked goal can bring on a feeling of hopelessness and helplessness.

Instead of focusing on what you cannot change, focus on what you can within the circumstance. You can't stop your loved one from dying, but you can make the rest of his/her living worthwhile, loved, and cherished.

There is always a positive. There is always another way to deal with what is going on in life. Choose to find it. Choose to put that positive at the end of the sentence and watch your emotions turn around. If you really find yourself stuck, you need to get help so that the depression does not steal your life. Hospice to the rescue again; they will provide you with counseling.

FEELING OVERWHELM AND EXHAUSTION

Caring for another person around the clock will definitely make you tired. Some nights might not hold much sleep, and some days seem endless. Your body can only take so much.

When I started to feel so tired that I felt sick, I called hospice. Mom was not sleeping well, and I was up several times a night with her. I asked them to speak with the doctor about the possibility of a sleeping pill for her. He would make the best decision based on her illness and medications. I then spoke with Mom and suggested to her that she use a sleeping pill if the doctor agreed. I knew that she had taken them in the past. She thought it would be very helpful. The doctor agreed, and that night we both got a full 6-7 hours of sleep.

If you are not getting rest and renewal, you will burn out and be of no help. What do you need? Is it more sleep? Do you need time off during the day? Would help around the house save some energy? Figure out what would be the most help, and then determine to have that need met.

LONELINESS

When you care for someone full time, going to lunch or coffee or a movie or just hanging out with a friend might not be possible. Day in and out, you find yourself alone. There becomes a routine of care between you and your loved one, but you probably need more.

While friends and family are often there at the beginning, they have lives of their own and tend to return to them. This can leave you feeling very alone. Do something about it.

Arrange to get out with friends or to go shopping or play a round of golf. Whatever helps you. It is not selfish or uncaring to do this. Do not feel guilty about taking care of yourself. You will return with more energy, a better mood, and renewed vitality. You will return better able to take care of your loved one.

If you just can't get out, then call someone. You can also text, email, or join a social network. Do not assume that you have to be alone or that you can do nothing about loneliness.

FEAR AND ANXIETY

You also might experience fear and anxiety. Learning about your loved one's disease and its course can help to ease the fear. Later in the book, we will talk about what to expect as death approaches. It is hard to watch for these signs, but knowing what is to come alleviates anxiety.

You are learning and becoming equipped to care. You are finding out the "how to" that fills in the blanks of your knowledge of caring. Preparation can take away much fear and help as you move to the future.

If you feel that fear and anxiety are getting a foothold, then call hospice and see about getting some counseling help. Don't wait too long.

ANGER

Anger can be a part of grief, and grief is about loss. You may find that you have a **loss of independence** and that you are angry about it. Well, yes it is probably true, but it is temporary. This is an opportunity for you to grow like few who come your way. **Rather than focus on what you can't do— focus on what you can become.**

You might have a **loss of friends** and be angry with them. In times like these, you begin to learn more about those closest to you. You will see their strengths and weaknesses. Be gentle with them. Put yourself in their shoes. What would you be doing? Would you know what to say or how to help? Would you feel in the way or completely useless in the situation?

Think of what emotions the situation might be bringing up in them. Did they recently lose someone? Is this potentially triggering their grief? Does this cause them to fear their own mortality? Are you seeing an area of immaturity or lack of commitment in them?

Yes, this hurts. With those you can, tell them that you miss them and that you are hurt. With those you can't, write a letter to them that you don't intend to send. After you have written it, destroy it. Getting the anger up and out of you is very helpful. Write as many letters as you need to. Just remember to always destroy them afterward.

Find other safe ways to express your anger. One of the best ways is talking with a safe person. This could be a friend, family member, or counselor. Anger often covers hurt. See if there is hurt underneath that needs to be addressed. Just talking can often help you to understand what is going on inside you and help you to deal with it.

HELPLESS

You can't change the course of the journey. You must continue until the end. It is hard to watch someone you love deteriorate. It is hard to watch them die. But you are not helpless.

You have the power to love. You have the capacity to care. You can do the only thing that matters—treat another human being as the amazing, precious, fragile, loved-of-God person that s/he is. You will look back on this time and know that you made a difference.

RESENTMENT

This again, has to do with loss. The illness stole the future you may have had planned and you resent it. You may need more help. Yet those who should help aren't, and you resent it. You may resent caregiving, not having your freedom, and losing the normality of your life.

Some resentment might be a normal part of grief, but it can quickly turn into bitterness. If this is happening to you, please get some help. Bitterness will eat you alive, hurts everyone around you, and steals your life. You will look back and realize what you lost by being bitter.

Forgive where you can. Accept life as it is for you now. Let go of what you wanted life to be and start seeing what you can do with the new life that is now yours. Be focused on the future rather than obsessing about what could or should have been.

GUILT

Guilt can be real and imagined. Guilt means that you did something wrong and you feel it inside and can do something about it—make it right. But what if you didn't actually do anything wrong? Feeling guilty doesn't produce anything of value then.

It is normal to want this ordeal to end. It is normal to want to get back to your life. It is also normal to feel guilty for thinking these things. You wonder how you could have such thoughts while your loved one is dying. It's not that you want them to go; it is that this is hard, and you want it to end.

You may get the opportunity to go out with friends and then feel guilty about having a great time. It is okay to still be alive and to smell the roses along the way. You would probably prefer that your loved one was well and able to have the same opportunities.

Unless you have actually done something wrong, then please try to control these thoughts. Laughing, crying, hoping, and sadness are all part of life. Just live—it's okay to do so.

INSECURE AND OUT OF CONTROL

In some ways, you are at the mercy of the winds and tides on this journey. It will end when you arrive, and you just have to let it take you where it will. The only control you actually have is over yourself and what you do as you drift.

Skills can be learned, and you can be in charge of those things over which you actually have control. Reading this book is helping you learn some skills so that you feel less insecure. Figuring out where you actually have control and then doing what you can will give you a sense of purpose on this passage.

GRIEF

Grief is your companion at each stage along the journey. Grief comes immediately upon the news that a cure is not possible. This grief continues past the funeral and possibly for years to come.

We will talk more about grief later in the book. For now, just know that with each change in your loved one's health, there is more grief. When they can no longer walk, there is a loss. When it becomes difficult to eat or drink, you will feel loss again. We lose our loved ones in stages. So each stage brings new feelings of grief.

Know that what you feel is normal. Rather than trying to stuff it down or deny it, notice it, allow it, and feel it. Grief is your companion, and you can learn from it and grow from it.

STAYING AWAY FROM THE MONSTERS OF THE DEEP

Emotions feel as if they can capsize the ship. They certainly can make you feel off balance. But there are some ways to maintain stability.

1. **Keep a journal**: Think of them as log entries on the journey. This very book is written because I kept a journal while my mother was here with me. Having a safe place to write my thoughts and feelings helped me to process. It also became a record of my time with her. Even now, I re-read it and realize that I had forgotten some things that happened. I am so glad I can look back now. You can read it at the end of this book.

2. **Watch your self-talk**: Listen to what is going on between your ears. Is it very negative or hopeless? Are you remembering to add in some positives? The battle is always here in the mind. Take control of what you are thinking and watch your emotions change.

3. **Stay close to God**: Talk with Him even if what you have to say is angry. He can handle your anger. Just talk to Him. This time will test what you really believe and help you to examine your faith. I wish I could tell you why things are happening as they are. All I can say is that I have faith in the character of God and trust that He knows what He is doing and has a plan. Try to see your circumstances through His eyes rather than see Him through your circumstances.

4. **Respite**: You might need to take a quick port of call. Sometimes you just need time off in order to regroup, rest, and recuperate so that you can jump back in. Do it when you need to.

5. **Coping strategies:** In addition to what we have talked about so far, here are a few more strategies to help you cope and thrive.
    - *Laughter:* They say it is a good medicine. And it is. Watch a really funny movie or find something else that makes you laugh. It is more than okay to have a bit of entertainment and fun. It will even brighten your mood and remind you that not all of life is serious or tragic.
    - *Talk with friends and family*: Converse with people who are safe and supportive. Let yourself connect with others. Ask about their lives, too. That way you can have a porthole of sorts; you can see outside the current events in your life.
    - *Develop a network of help*. This can be on the Internet, in person, by mail, etc. Look for home or community-based programs that help with homemaking or meals, that provide legal or financial counsel. There are a lot of resources out there. If you don't have time to look for them, ask a friend or family member to find what you need. It is okay to need help.
    - *Organize:* Decluttering and organizing brings a sense of peace while clutter and disorganization adds to stress. Take 15 minutes at a time to work on an area. Set a timer. You don't have to do it all at once. We eat an elephant one bite at a time.

- *Join a support group:* This can be an in-person or an Internet community. Either way, it will have in it people who share your experience. They understand what you feel. Others may say that they know how you feel but these people really do.

6. **Transferring your loved one to a hospice facility**. There may come a time when it is too much for you. Your health—mental, emotional and physical—might be at risk. Making the decision to move to a facility from your home does not mean that you are abandoning your loved one. It means that the primary care will belong to another so that you can spend your time with your loved one loving, talking, and caring for him/her differently.

   This decision might be very difficult, and you may also have to deal with what others' might think of your decision. Remember, they are not in your shoes and can't understand. You can listen to their opinions, but at the end of the day you have to do what is right for you and your loved one.

When you are far from shore and far from your destination it can be a bit scary. But, you can take steps to care for yourself and your loved one. Ultimately there is peace and love after you work through all these fears and concerns.

Take your time, listen to your heart and your loved one, and take steps to keep the monsters at bay.

CHAPTER SEVEN WORKBOOK

Your loved one's "monsters" ______________________________

____

____

____

____

____

____

____

____

____

____

Your "monsters" ______________________________________

____

____

____

____

____

____

____

____

____

____

Rate your self-talk

1 2 3 4 5 6 7 8 9 10

Negative Positive

Coping strategies I will use... ______________________________

Who I will talk with about this journey... ______________________________

JOURNAL

How I am dealing with the fear of monsters and steering clear of them...

Chapter Eight

APPROACHING THE HORIZON AND LOOKING BACK

Life can only be understood backward, but it must be lived forward
~Soren Kierkegaard

As you near the horizon, your loved one will be thinking more and more about his/her past. Your loved one is looking backwards at his/her journey, taking inventory, looking for meaning, and asking questions.

There are some very specific needs at this time with which you can help your loved one. **What does your loved one need to finish well?**

CLOSURE

Your loved one needs closure of **worldly concerns.** S/he will want to know what will happen with the things they have accumulated and the debts that she might owe. Help your loved one finish legal, financial, and material issues.

Your loved one will also seek closure with **relationships**. S/he might be thinking of loss, forgiveness to give, and forgiveness needed to receive. Your loved one will be concerned with those left behind. Those relationships that still have unresolved issues will be of major focus.

You may not think of this, but your loved one will need closure with his/her **community**. This will include work, friends, groups, church, etc.

MEANING

As people approach their death they might wonder, "Did it matter that I walked this earth?" They want to know that their lives had meaning. They want to know if they made an impact on both the world in general and within their personal history.

ACCEPTANCE

The last stage in grief is acceptance. As your loved one finds closure and meaning in reviewing his/her life, your loved one will start to become ready to end his/her days here. The hope is that your loved one accepts death and has made peace with his/her life history, relationships and role on the earth. Some people, unfortunately, die bitter and angry. They accept that they are dying, but they take a lack of forgiveness and regrets to their graves.

A woman I know talked bitterly about her ex-husband who had divorced her some forty years earlier the day before she died. How tragic that she could not forgive him and that this resentment was still eating at her soul after so many years. She did not die in peace.

A truly peaceful passage where one lets go of life here comes about after there is closure. The person finds that life had meaning and finds acceptance, forgiveness, and grace.

LOVE

Maybe the Beatles were right when they said, "love is all you need." At this time of life when all is said and done, all that really matters is the love we give and receive. The things one has accumulated are not as important as those moments of love remembered. And until the very last breath, love is still available to give and receive.

Give lavishly. Receive heartily.

HOW TO HELP YOUR LOVED ONE FINISH WELL

Help your loved one to tell his/her story: They want to have purpose in these last days rather than just wait to die. Helping your loved one to tell the story of his/her life will allow them to feel that they are passing on what they have learned to the generations to come.

Your loved one can tell of times focused on what s/he now finds matters little so that you can learn to focus on what really matters today. Your loved one can tell you of what s/he did really well and how s/he has found peace and forgiveness for what s/he did not.

As your loved one tells their story and reviews his/her life, your loved one will find that s/he really did make an impact and truly affected those around him/her. Your loved one will learn that it mattered that s/he walked this earth.

Help your loved one to come to closure: This means closure with the people, events, and possessions in your loved one's life. Let your loved one know that his/her wishes for the estate will be handled as s/he wishes. Listen to his/her concerns and hurts, joys and accomplishments in the events of your loved one's days. Facilitate closure by helping your loved one contact those s/he wishes to speak with or see before s/he goes.

Help your loved one to remember: It is important that your loved one remember how much s/he has been through and handled well. Even what went very wrong in your loved one's life was most likely a time of great personal growth. Ask questions about what s/he learned, how s/he grew. Help your loved one to find those precious gems among the mundane and difficult.

How your loved one processes this will be a reflection of his/her temperament. If your loved one is the artistic type, you might want to provide a favorite way of expression. If your loved one is more the academic or structured person, you might want to write down a chronological history. Honor who your loved one is in this process.

Help your loved one to forgive: Lack of forgiveness toward oneself or others is a debtor's prison. The weight of the debt weighs on one without relief. Only forgiveness brings peace.

Forgiveness is the transference of a debt—much like a mortgage that is sold to a different bank. You still owe the debt, just not to the original debtor. To forgive is to take the debt that another owes you (emotional, physical, financial, etc.) and give it to God. The "debtor" is still on the hook, just not on yours.

We serve a just God and He will know what to do with this debt. It might be that He allows the consequences of the debtor's actions to play out in his/her life. It might be that He gives it to His Son to take to the cross. The point is, one who forgives is freed from the debt and has its weight removed.

There are several types of people you and your loved one should forgive:

- anyone with whom you still hold a grudge
- yourself
- God

I know it sounds strange to forgive God, but many people feel that He has hurt them or not been there for them. They allow this to come between them and God. God cannot do wrong, so it is your loved one's perception or lack of understanding that causes him/her to believe God owes him/her a debt.

As you help your loved one to review his/her past, you will be giving your loved one a gift. In this way, your loved one can move onto a new life and become a new person.

CHAPTER EIGHT WORKBOOK

Where you can help your loved with closure:

- Worldly possessions and goods ______________________

- Relationships ______________________

- Community ______________________

How I can help my loved one tell his/her story... ______________________

Here is how I will be ready to talk with my loved one about forgiveness... ______________________

JOURNAL

As I think of my own meaning and story... ____________________

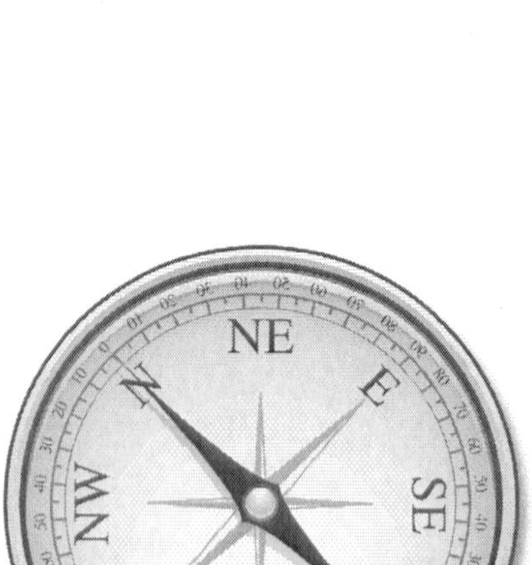
N
NE
E
SE
S
SW
W
NW

Chapter Nine

COURSE CORRECTIONS: FINDING YOURSELF IN THE JOURNEY

When your heart speaks, take good notes.

~Judith Campbell

Before your loved one came to this final passage, you were continuing your daily routine. You had plans and a schedule, friends and family. Now, all that is on hold as you take this passage with your loved one. Caregiving itself changes your course and alters your life.

This major change in your daily life may leave you feeling lost. You might feel numb or not know what you feel anymore as you are ripped from your comfort zone and thrust into this journey. But, this journey will actually help you **find your way back to yourself**: a new, improved self.

Being out of your comfort zone will stretch you, test you, and help you to grow. You will find resources inside yourself that you didn't know you had and would not have found had you not been placed on this journey. Rather than try to hold onto who you have been, you have to let go and travel with the current—wherever it will take you.

This is a sailboat not a motorboat. You have to go where the wind blows and it varies much like the ebbing and flowing of the tide. Some days will feel like you are moving quickly and others will feel as if time is standing still. There will be days that you believe you are stretched to your limit, and others where you feel strong and competent and ready for anything.

Within this journey are lessons to learn.

You can learn to love even deeper and better than you ever have. Love is a choice. Love chooses to do what is best for the beloved. It thinks of ways to show itself.

You have the opportunity to learn to serve others rather than be the center of your universe. Serving another means that sometimes you have to put someone else first. It requires a humbling of yourself so that you can help another in their need.

You are not a victim unless you choose to be. If the whole experience is about you then you could certainly end up with a victim mentality. You will be thinking "poor me" and "look what I have to put up with and do" rather than choosing to focus. Remember, you are providing a peaceful, loving passage for you and your loved one by serving them.

You can learn to not only face your emotions, but see them as part of your humanity. You will not be ruled by them. Your weakness, frailty, pain, and fear will all rise to the surface during this time. They all indicate that you are part of the human race. We all feel these things at times. It is okay for you to feel them, as well.

Give yourself grace. Be patient with yourself. Feel what you feel, but don't give up. As you keep moving forward, despite a storm within, you will learn to handle intense emotion. You will find that you are not crushed as you feared you might be. You can continue on even with loss. It is possible to thrive under stressful times.

When you look back, you will recognize that you really did a good job with little training, ever-changing circumstances, and constant heartache.

You can learn to stop isolating and protecting your heart and risk letting others see who you really are. We used to tell each other to be tough, suck it up, and stop crying when times were hard. What that did was force our humanity underground. We felt that it was not okay to cry; we felt that crying somehow made us weak.

Letting others (those safe people in your life) see what you are feeling is actually an invitation to a deeper relationship. If you risk showing your heart, and it is seen as the precious, vulnerable, fragile, and wonderful thing that it is and is treated that way—then you have now reached a more intimate friendship than ever. You gave someone else the gift of your true self. If they honor that, then this is a companion worth having. If they do not, then move on and find another person who is worthy of your time, affections, and heart.

You can learn to stop being controlled by others' guilt tripping and be responsible for and to yourself. If you live to please everyone, then you will please no one—especially yourself and God. Many people will try to suck you into their world. In that world you, and everyone else, is supposed to act as they see fit, speak, say, and feel as they would dictate.

These are the ones who will tell you what you "should" do, what you "can't" do, and attempt to make you feel guilty for being, thinking, or feeling anything of which they do not approve. If you comply, then you have just given them the power to determine who you will be.

This is where **boundaries** come in.

A boundary says, "This is who I am, what I think, what I feel, what I want, and what I don't want." A boundary simply defines who you are. You are not an extension of anyone else (regardless of what they say). You are free to be you; they are free to be them. When people place their "shoulds" on you, they are showing disrespect for you as an individual. In your mind simply say, "No agreement."

"No, I don't agree that I have to do this the way you are trying to force me to."

"No, I don't agree that I should feel the way that you say I should."

"No, I don't agree that you have the right to control my life."

Here is the key: when you feel pressure from others, go to the Lord and ask Him what He thinks. If He is fine with who you are and how you are handing things, then it does not matter what anyone else thinks. But go humbly willing to hear that you are incorrect and that it would benefit you to listen to what they are saying.

The point is, be responsible for and to yourself before God—and let others do the same.

You can learn to be where your feet are: Being where your feet are means that you live not in the past or future but right now, right where you are. When we live in the past or what might or could happen, we miss the moments we own right now. This is one reason forgiveness is so important—it releases us from the past so we can live today.

When you are living in the present you are not thinking so much of the life you had before the illness or how it will be after it is over. Instead, you are fully in the day, fully in your emotions, and fully with your loved ones.

Your loved one is still with you. Yes, your loved one is moving toward death but s/he is still alive up until that moment. You don't have to fear what is not present; you have to deal with what is right before you. The illness is not the center of the universe. What matters is the life and love we do with one another right now.

UNFINISHED BUSINESS

Within this journey, you will find that you need to make further course corrections. Unfinished business in your relationship with your dying loved one will rise to the surface and demand your attention.

If your dying loved one is a parent, you will find yourself revisiting your childhood growing up with them. Unresolved issues may have been pushed below the surface, but they will be very present now. Old hurts, resentments, jealousies, and the repressed unsaid will all rise for you to feel and deal with.

At first, this may seem like a horrible time to have to handle these issues. In truth, now is the perfect time to deal with these issues, precisely because you need to deal with them.

To be able to give and receive forgiveness with your loved one while they are still here is very healing. If you don't do this now, after your loved one is gone you may feel like there is no way to find the closure you need.

In the last chapter, we talked about **forgiveness** as transference of a debt. You gather up all that you believe the other owes you (the hurts, losses, etc.) and give them over to God. The debt now belongs to Him. You will find that if you do this on your own, when you are with your loved one later you have far less hurt or resentment or pain.

Once you forgive, you are freer to love—the debt no longer stands between you or feels like an elephant in the room. You will also need to forgive yourself for any problems in the relationship with your loved one.

When this is done, it will be easier to speak with your loved one about any issue that you still feel needs some dialogue.

FINDING BALANCE

The way your life balanced prior to your loved one beginning this passage is no longer applicable. That does not mean that balance is not possible. It means that it will just be a bit more difficult until you get your sea legs.

You will see a new rhythm in your life. Don't look for each day to balance out, but that you find that balance between caregiving, family, work, finances, etc. over a longer stretch of time. Some days you may not be able to get much done other than loving and caring. Stay present in that. Other days you will be able to attend to many tasks and find that you are able to get a remarkable amount accomplished. And, some days you will find that rest is most needed. Do what you can, when you can, and I promise it will all even out in the end.

YOU WILL FIND YOU IN THIS JOURNEY

You won't come out of this journey the same person as you were when you started. You will come out of this as more than you knew you were or could be. Stay present, learn to love, and set boundaries. Feel what you feel and serve your way to a new you.

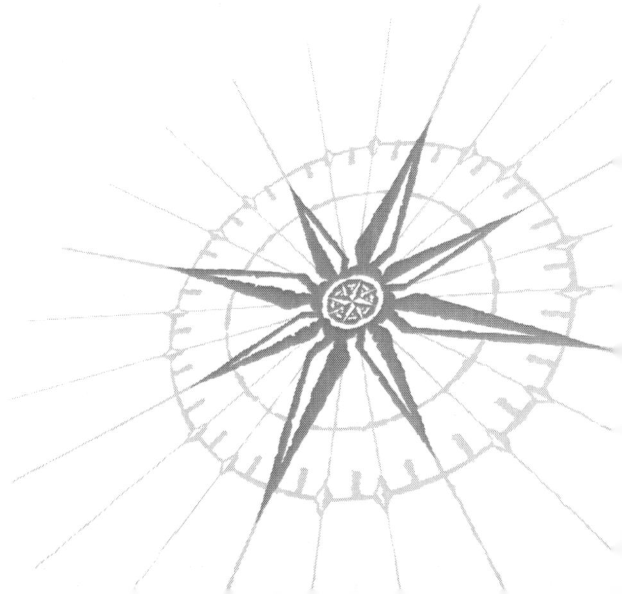

CHAPTER NINE WORKBOOK

Where do you love deeper and better? ______________________

____

____

____

____

____

How are you at serving? ______________________________

____

____

____

____

____

Are you facing your emotions or running? Why or why not?

____

____

____

____

____

Where are you protecting rather than risking? ______________

____

____

____

____

____

Who is trying to control you, and how will you set boundaries with them?

When are you least in the moment?

What is your unfinished business and where do you still need to forgive?

JOURNAL

I am changing...

Chapter Ten

THE NORTH STAR WILL GUIDE YOU

I have been driven many times to my knees by the overwhelming conviction that I had nowhere else to go.

~Abraham Lincoln

Coming to the end of one's life or being with someone who is will undoubtedly bring up thoughts of God. Even if there has been little in the pursuit of God throughout life there will at least be the consideration of the possibility of His existence on this journey.

A RITE OF PASSAGE

As your loved one reviews his/her life your loved one will begin to wonder and ponder about the one to come. Closure in this life makes possible a peaceful passage to the next.

WHERE AM I GOING?

Many people have a belief in a higher power that oversees their lives and cares for them. These people start their final journey with a destination in mind. Knowing where you are going and trusting the process to God brings peace and calm. They end their lives ready for the next.

Some people had a belief at an earlier time in life, moved away from it, and now will start to revisit it. The things that took up their time and thoughts will soon no longer be part of their lives. The energy spent accumulating possessions seems less important as all of those things must be left behind. Even the relationships they cherished are about to end. And there, coming forward, are memories of Bible stories and going to church and, suddenly, they do seem more important.

Some people never gave it much thought or had no belief in an afterlife at all. There is a very good chance that they will be considering it now. What if they are wrong and there really is a God? Will they be ready to meet Him? Will He accept them if they rejected Him their whole lives? What if He really exists and does love them? What if they could meet Him right now just by asking to?

SPIRITUALLY THIRSTY

Even if your loved one or you have never been thirsty for the spiritual before, you likely will be at least thinking about it now. Here, at this time, one begins to realize that life here on earth is not all there is. There is more to the picture. This thirst will demand to be satisfied.

Your loved one may feel guilt as s/he thinks back on the wrongs done. You can tell your loved one that there is forgiveness awaiting him/her. Your loved one simply has to ask.

Your loved one may wonder what God is like. You can tell him/her that Jesus walked the earth so that we could look at him and see who God is: generous, compassionate, loving, truthful, humble, forgiving and inviting.

Your loved one may question whether s/he can have peace with God. You can tell your loved one that Jesus came so that s/he could have peace. He died for every wrong people ever did and so, your loved one is not guilty if s/he accepts that he took on his/her punishment.

This is my belief system, and it was also my mother's. From the moment she was told that she would not live, she had peace. In the time I cared for her, I never saw fear of what was to come. As she got closer to death the only one she said she wanted to talk with was God. She died in peace because she believed in God and that she was going to be with Him.

WHAT WAS GOD DOING IN YOUR LOVED ONE'S LIFE?

So, what then was life all about?

Think back on geometry and the idea of the "line segment." It starts with a point, an origin, and then continues on forever. The point, the dot, is your life here on earth. It is the shortest part of your life. This time on earth, whether short or long, is only the tiny dot that starts the line that goes on forever. This time here prepares us for forever.

I believe that God will give us what we want. It's called "free-will."

If we want Him, if we choose to believe in Him and follow Him, then He is what we get for eternity. Since He is all good, all love, He is light without darkness, then that goodness and love and light will be our forever experience.

If we don't want Him or don't accept Him, then forever we will experience the absence of God in our eternal lives. That means no good, no love, no light—forever.

In this short part of our lives we make a choice that then goes on without end. So, all of our lives here are about making a choice that God will grant us.

Your loved one's life, like all of ours, is about making a decision for or against God. At this time of their lives they will be thinking about this decision more and more.

TESTED FAITH

"Who do you say that I am?" That is the question that God asks all of us. In this final journey, that question must be answered.

In these last days, paradigms about God that don't match up with who He actually is come forward. Questions of fairness and "why" arise. However, God often wants us to trust that He is who He says that He is and have faith and, so, does not answer our questions. That tests faith but also refines it.

SOMETIMES THERE IS ANGER AT GOD

Fear can produce anger.
Anger can make one feel powerful at a time when one feels so helpless. Getting mad makes that fear move to the background for a time and gives a feeling of some control.

Not wanting to let go can produce anger.
Leaving the world behind is difficult. There are people, places, and things that have been loved. There are memories that hold one here and possibilities that make one not want to depart. Being forced to give all that up can bring anger.

Not understanding Him can produce anger.
Why me? Why now? Not understanding what He is doing and why can make one frustrated, angry, and demanding of an answer. Sometimes God does not answer. This brings one back to faith. Who do you say that He is? Is He trustworthy even when understanding isn't there? His character does not change and one must find comfort in this when the answers are missing.

We have to pray with our eyes on God, not on the difficulties.
~Oswald Chambers

ACCEPTANCE

Trusting in God, faith, brings thankfulness for life and even acceptance. Accepting that this is part of His plan, trusting in His character, and believing that He has a plan for all settles the soul and brings peace.

You will see your loved one come to a place of calm and tranquility when s/he is prepared and ready. Your loved one may get there before you. Your loved one has struggled with God, reviewed his/her life and found closure and s/he will prepare for the horizon.

WHAT IS GOD DOING IN YOU ON THIS JOURNEY

You will find yourself confronted with your own humanity on this journey. The fact that one day you will find yourself facing the end of your own life becomes very clear as you take this final journey with another.

Your own faith will be tested. You might find that you have anger at God and that you are struggling with who He is and why He is doing this. This is a time of tremendous spiritual growth for you and your loved one.

> *If you seek me with all of your heart, I will be found by you says the Lord God Almighty.*

This is a time of seeking after God. You can find Him, find His comfort, strength, and presence.

Be with God during the changes that He is causing in you—your spiritual growth. He will be your anchor, keeping you safe through this storm. He will get you through this. You are not alone; He is with you even when you are angry with Him.

Practice His presence.
Throughout your day, remind yourself that He is right there with you. This is not prayer. It is just knowing that whatever you do, He is with you. Then, when you do need to turn to Him, you will find Him ready and waiting to help.

It is said that God doesn't give you more than you can handle. I don't believe that. I believe that He doesn't give you more than HE can handle. If you are trying to make this journey without Him, you may find that the weight of this is too much for you. With Him, you will find that He takes the majority of the weight onto His own shoulders and remains there with you to love you, weep with you, and even give you joy.

Being with God moment by moment is where we learn how to be ourselves, and it gives life its unique flavor and significance. With Him you are always loved, always significant, always safe, always valued, and never alone.

Taking this journey with Him **you will be transformed**. The process is a mirror showing you a lot about yourself and giving you opportunities to change.

In this time, you will see your strength like never before. You will see your weaknesses, and rather than turn away, you can now see them as opportunities for growth.

You are human: give yourself grace as you are stretched and grown. Accept who you are now but know that God is not done with you. This journey is part of His plan to mature you and help you become who He always intended you to be.

As He walks with you through this time, you will **see your capacity to love increased**. Since God is love, being with Him enables you to love more. **Serving** the one who is dying in your home is easier from a heart of love. The small tasks that you do in this way will mean a lot to your loved one. Jesus did the lowly task of washing His disciples' feet, and they loved Him all the more. You will do many lowly tasks as you care for your loved one. Performing these tasks from a place of love will inspire your loved one and may push them to open up more, as well.

We take this journey with God. He is in the details with you doing His part. All you need to do is stay by His side, do what needs to be done, and find that all of this draws you closer to Him and gives you peace.

CHAPTER TEN WORKBOOK

How can you help your loved one with their spiritual concerns?

What is God doing in you?

JOURNAL

Dear God...

Chapter Eleven

MAKING LAND WHILE THEY SAIL ON

When you were born, you cried and the world rejoiced. Live your life in such a manner that when you die the world cries and you rejoice.
~Indian Saying

At this point in the journey, time is suddenly speeding up. You are nearing the end. There is a sense of waiting in expectation, yet you feel that time is hurrying along.

Every journey has an end, and you have been sailing toward this port. All your work, all your sacrifice was for this time. You have been working toward a peaceful passage.

You have done a good job even when you made mistakes. It is about the heart, and you have undertaken a journey with your loved one that many never will. You were called upon to go into unexpected and uncharted territories feeling badly equipped and wholly inadequate for the task. The journey with your loved one is just about over.

You have done what you could do, and now you have to let go so that your loved one can continue on.

THE ENDING OF THE JOURNEY

You will remember these last days and last moments intensely. Many of the tasks and days will blend together but this end of the journey you will remember.

You may feel anxious or afraid to speak, but I want to encourage you to be authentic; I want you to say what needs to be said. These last days can be very intimate or at least will be very heart-engaged.

Your emotions will be intense and varied. You may feel that you are on a roller coaster or on pins and needles. You wait for the last breath and dread it all at the same time. Will it be in the next minutes or days?

This is a sacred time. You are accompanying your loved one to the end of life here and the beginning of a new life. *This mortal must put on immortality.* And you are here just as that happens.

Let your loved one know you will be there, that you will stay. When everything is said and done, all that will be left is love.

LET YOUR LOVED ONE GO

Sometimes people need permission to go on. Tell your loved one that s/he can leave—it is okay—you will be okay. Let your loved one know that you will keep vigil until s/he has gone.

Make sure your loved one knows that you will not forget him/her and that you will continue to love him/her. Tell your loved one that you want his/her suffering to end, for them to leave this dying body and that you will see him/her again.

PHYSICAL CHANGES AT THE END

Death and dying is a process, and although there are some similarities with every passing—they are not the same. You can watch for signs but know that you may not see all of them. Stay present and attend to your loved one and his/her needs at each stage.

Even if your loved one doesn't know that you are there, you can sit with him/her and just stay present. You can touch your loved one if it is not uncomfortable.

MONTHS OUT

Disconnecting from life and going inward to process.

- Conversation with others lessens. Your loved one might want less company, less television, or less music. Your loved one seems to be thinking and processing something. This is part of the reviewing of life. Be available to listen or talk as needed.

- Your loved one might want to be alone more often. This is not a rejection of you or others but, again, part of your loved one processing the meaning of their life before moving on.

Changes in appetite.

- Your loved one will usually want less to eat and drink; this is part of dying—the body is shutting down and needs less. This can be difficult for you, and you may feel the need to force fluids or food. Just remember, this change is normal.

Changes in urination and bowels.

- These functions are slowing down as the need for food and fluids also diminishes. The body is beginning to slow down.

Sleeping more.

- Your loved one may seem to sleep more than usual. Naps become more frequent and nighttime sleeping may become heavier, as well.

WEEKS OUT

Sleeping even more but can be awakened.

- Your loved one may begin to sleep a good portion of the day. Naps are frequent, but if you move or speak to your loved one s/he awakens only to go back to sleep.

Conversations with someone you can't see.

- This is not an uncommon experience. A nurse friend was visiting one day when we watched my Mom talking with someone we couldn't see. She seemed to be getting instructions, saying, "okay…yes…okay." My friend said that when this happened in the hospital, the staff wrote it out in red in the chart as it meant the patient was nearing death.

Agitation.

- Your loved one may appear restless and unable to get comfortable. You might see your loved one pulling or picking at clothes or bedding.

- Check on your loved one's pain level and give medication as needed. If your loved one's agitation is due to pain, this can be alleviated.

Confusion.

- Your loved one may not know where s/he is, the day of the week, or even who you are. As the body is shutting down, there will be changes that could effect the body and mind. Be patient, calm, and helpful.

They want to go on a trip.

- Many people will try to get out of bed or ask to have their bags packed. They are getting ready to leave and feel the impulse to get ready to go.

Skin color might flush or be bluish.

- If there is a fever present, the skin will be rosier. If less oxygen is getting to the extremities, the skin will begin to look blue.

Breathing may change.

- You may notice that your loved one's breathing is faster or slower than usual, even changing rhythm or pausing.

Body temperature can fluctuate.

- Your loved one might experience fever, sweating, or chills.
- You may notice increased perspiration.

Congestion and coughing.

- It may be that your loved one begins to have fluid in the lungs that cause coughing.

Symptoms can come and go.

- One day your loved one may seem to be having many symptoms and the next very few. Symptoms can also come and go within the day.

Changes in appetite and fluid intake continue.

- Appetite continues to diminish, and your loved one might not want as many fluids.

DAYS OUT

Everything above now intensifies.

- As your loved one nears the end, the symptoms will become even more pronounced.

Your loved one can have a surge of energy, even getting up.

- Your loved one may suddenly feel fine and want to get up.
- Your loved one may want to eat a meal with you, sit up, or chat.
- Your loved one may even have the energy for an outing.

Irregular breathing continues.

- You will notice that your loved one's breathing is losing its rhythm or stopping only to start again.
- Death rattle" – is distressing to hear but, like snoring, the person is not aware of it nor is it painful to them.

Blood pressure and pulse are hard to find.

- As the body shuts down, less blood will go to your loved one's extremities, making it difficult to get a blood pressure reading or to feel a pulse.

Restlessness.

- Your loved one cannot get comfortable.
- Your loved one pulls at clothes or bedding.
- Your loved one moves continuously and may moan.
  - Check on pain levels and administer medications as needed.

Unconsciousness.

- Your loved one may no longer be able to be awakened.

Hands, feet, and knees become purple and blotchy, colder.

- Circulation begins to lessen or cease in extremities. The body is trying to keep the major organs going.

Eyes can become glassy and half open.

- Even though your loved one may not be conscious, his/her eyes might be slightly open.
- As you look at your loved one's eyes, they look glassy and do not focus on things around them.

Urine will decrease, but your loved one may wet or defecate in the bed.

- As the kidneys shut down, there may be much less urine.
- Your loved one might suddenly become incontinent even though they have not been before.
- Your loved one may have a stool in the bed.

Your loved one can still hear you, so speak from your heart.

- It is thought that the last sense to go is hearing.
- Though my mother had been seemingly unconscious all day when my daughter and her husband came, she responded and knew they were there.

MINUTES

Can't be awakened.

There is no longer any response to his/her surroundings

Might be a sudden convulsion.

- A shudder or convulsion might happen. This can be very disturbing to watch, but your loved one is most likely in no pain.

Might yell or spasm.

- As breathing changes and death approaches, there might be a moan or yell. Again, this is most likely not due to pain but caused by a spasm.

"Fish out of water" breathing.

- Breathing is very shallow and rapid with the mouth open.

Breathing stops only to have another breath after a long wait.

- You may think that your loved one has passed only to have them take another breath after a very long pause.

DEATH

Heartbeat and breathing stop.

- When this happens, your loved one has passed.

Eyes are usually open at least slightly.

- Despite what the movies portray, the eyes are usually not closed. You may leave your loved one as s/he is, or you can close the eyes.

Mouth will probably be relaxed and slightly open.

- The mouth is usually not closed. Again, if this bothers you, it might be possible to close your loved one's mouth.

Skin color pales.

- As oxygen is no longer coming into the body, it will begin to pale and mottle.

There is a sense that your loved one is no longer present.

- Although your loved one's body is still here, your loved one is gone. Your loved one has moved out much like when we move from one home to another. You have witnessed an eternal transition.

The end of a very long journey with your loved one has ended. This is a very precious, sacred, life-changing time for you and you can stay here with your loved one for awhile.

It is okay to feel whatever you feel.
You may feel relief that it is over.
You may feel happy for your loved one.
You may feel grief overtake you, and all you can do is weep.

All your loving and serving your loved one as s/he moved toward this destination is just about over. Although you cannot see your loved one now, s/he still lives. Your loved one has moved from your loving arms into the arms of the One who loves them.

There is just a bit more to do.

CHAPTER ELEVEN WORKBOOK

What keeps you for letting your loved one go? ________________

Who does your loved one want near as s/he approaches the end of his/her journey? ________________

Who do you need there to support you? ________________

JOURNAL

As my loved one approaches death... ______________________

Chapter Twelve

FINISHING UP THE JOURNEY

Every day is an opportunity to make a new happy ending.

~Author Unknown

AFTER THE DEATH

Stay with your loved one's body if you want for as long as you want. There is no hurry. You can sit with the now empty body and talk awhile or just sit quietly. Maybe family members would like to be there, and you can comfort one another.

Don't be rushed; take this precious time. Some may want to push you through this stage; don't let it happen. You won't want to stay here forever and a few minutes or more are perfectly fine.

This may be the only opportunity you get to say goodbye quietly before the funeral. Your loved one is truly gone, and you can begin to find some closure in these moments.

Others might want to do the same. Maybe you have some family or friends who would like to come and say their goodbyes. Be sure to give those who loved your loved one time alone if they need it.

You can clean or dress your loved one if you want. My daughter wanted to wash Mom's face and hands, and I watched her do so with tenderness and respect. It was part of her goodbye process.

WHO YOU CALL AND WHAT HAPPENS NEXT

It is best to call your Hospice organization. A nurse will come and confirm the death and start the paperwork. Our nurse sat with Mom's body until the funeral home arrived. The family went in the other room to care for one another, and it was good to know Mom was not alone.

By now, you will have given Hospice the information on the mortuary you picked. They will call for you, if you want. Let them do their job now while you take care of you.

The Hospice nurse will call the doctor for a death certificate. The nurse will also destroy all leftover medications for you and remove them from the home. Hospice will make sure that you and your family are okay and will ask if you would like a chaplain or counselor.

WHEN THE FUNERAL HOME COMES

Every mortuary has a different way that they care for the body. I assumed they would take my mother away in a body bag, but I did not want to see this. With this in mind, I initially decided against watching them remove the body.

I asked the nurse how they would treat the body, and she talked with the attendants for me. They said that family members should see a loved one leave with care and respect. When they brought Mom's body out of the room on the stretcher, she was covered with a beautiful blanket and her face looked as if she were asleep. I kissed her goodbye and watched them wheel her into the van. We waved until they turned the corner. The nurse left, and we were on our own.

MAKING THE CALLS

Friends and family want to be notified. You should have a list ready so you don't have to figure it out now. Hopefully, you have agreed on who is to make the calls.

With every call you will be exposed to the grief of those who hear the news. This can be very difficult, as you are already dealing with your own loss. However, it can also be healing to share the love you both felt.

AT THE MORTUARY

There will be a lot of questions and if you plan ahead this will not be so difficult. It is a lot to deal with unprepared. The following list can help make this a smoother and less painful process. The mortuary will want to know:

- Who has the legal responsibility to make decisions?
    - The mortuary might need siblings to also sign documents.
- Your loved one's full legal name.

- The date and place of your loved one's birth.
- Your loved one's social security number.
- Your loved one's military rank and serial number, if available or applicable.
- The name and birthplace of your loved one's parents.
- How many death certificates will you need?
    - Think through your loved one's finances and holdings and whether each will need a certificate to finalize the estate.
- A decision on cremation or burial.
- The location of the burial.
- Will there be a graveside service and date?
    - The mortuary will arrange this for you.
- Do you want a grave marker?
- Will an obituary be published? If so, who will write it?

COSTS

Costs for a burial and funeral can vary greatly. If you do your research before your loved one's death, you will not make emotional and costly decisions now.

Here are some of the expenses you may incur:

- Burial or cremation
    - Which best represents your loved one's wishes if they left no plan?
- Death certificates
- Casket or urn
    - These prices vary greatly. You don't have to buy these from the funeral home; you can find exactly what you need on-line these days.

- Chapel, church, or funeral home for the service
- Body transportation to the funeral and gravesite if cremation is not chosen
- Flowers
- Police escort if there are a large number of cars going from the funeral service to the gravesite
- Music for the funeral
- Pastor
- Cemetery plot
- Headstone
- Cemetery fees
    - mortuary will make these arrangements

TELLING YOUR LOVED ONE'S STORY

At the funeral you honor your loved one by remembering who s/he was, what your loved one did, and the impact s/he made on others. It is a celebration of your loved one's life and a grieving that s/he is gone.

Your loved one represented different roles to different people and, so, s/he is remembered differently. Perhaps your loved one was Mom or Dad, sister or brother, uncle, grandmother, or friend. There are many stories to be told of this person's different roles and relationships. It will be good to hear stories about your loved one. Your loved one's life impacted you, and now is the time to talk about how.

A funeral brings some closure. It is a public goodbye for the family and all who have been on this journey. Laughing and crying, talking about your loved one and telling his/her stories, helps to bring a finish to your loved one's days on earth. You remember that your loved one was here. Commemorate that life and take it forward in your memory now.

There is always a lot of emotion at a funeral. You will see and experience grief. There will be pain and laughter, talking and listening, and, hopefully, healing during this time.

The funeral is also a dedication to the future. It is a time to speak of the faith and hope of being reunited with your loved one someday. It is a looking back and a hope forward at the same time.

PLANNING THE FUNERAL

There are a lot of details to bring this celebration of their story to pass. Plan this as much ahead of time as possible. Your loved one may have had ideas of how they wanted to be remembered. Making their wishes happen now is a great way to honor them.

However, there are many details to attend to at a time of great grief. Grief can make us forgetful or make us feel foggy. So, here is a list of details you may need for the funeral.

- Will there be a memorial service and/or graveside service?
    - Can people come to both or will the graveside service be just for family?
- Is this a military funeral?
- Will there be a gathering after?
    - Where will it be held?

    - Will there be food, and who will provide it?
    - Do you need childcare?
        - Kids can draw or write a poem.
        - The children can still share memories and love.
        - Kids may be interested in writing letters to the deceased.
            - My daughter wrote a letter to her grandmother that was buried with the urn. It was her goodbye and helped her to heal.
- Who will help organize, set up, and clean up?
    - Delegate what you need.
- Will you need flowers and music?
    - Who will make arrangements for these?
- Who will officiate?
- Cemetery—burial, mausoleum, urn, scattered ashes?
- Pictures of the deceased.
    - Who will pick them and how will they be displayed?
- Travel and hotel for out of town guests.
    - Who will pick them up?
    - Where will they stay?

It is hard to grieve well when having to plan the funeral and all of the details that go with it. Hopefully, you have most of this planned ahead of time so that you can care for yourself and others when it is most needed.

CLOSING YOUR LOVED ONE'S ESTATE

When we leave this earth, we leave everything behind. For those of us who have lost our loved ones, we now see their shoes awaiting feet, their prized possessions just sitting there and a whole lot of work to do.

There are physical items, financial items, assets, and a whole list of people who must be contacted.

PACKING UP YOUR LOVED ONE'S THINGS

Putting away and distributing what our loved ones have left behind is hard. Thankfully, there is usually no hurry in getting this done. Sometimes the constant reminders of your loved one are comforting, and so keeping these items around a little while might actually be healing.

Family members might want to keep something that most reminds them of their loved one. Remember to honor the deceased's will, but giving these items to family members and friends can bring good memories to these people for years to come.

There are some aspects of estate closing that should be handled immediately. The will and trust documents should be read and the executor needs to start working on closing the estate.

The executor of the will makes sure that the assets are divided as the loved one wanted, creditors are paid, accounts closed, and the right agencies are notified. This might include:

- insurance providers—health, life, vehicle, and home
- employer benefits, such as a pension
- Social Security Agency (usually the funeral home notifies them of the death)
- banks, creditors, investment accounts, retirement accounts
- credit card companies
- utilities companies
- any other organization that might offer death benefits

You may also want to take care to do the following:

- forward mail to the executor
- cancel driver's license and change name on the titles of vehicles
- speak with the Veteran's Administration for possible benefits (if applicable)

All of this will be difficult. As you go through this, grief will be your ever-present companion. Let's talk about how to deal with it.

CHAPTER TWELVE WORKBOOK

List who is to be called after the death and who will make the calls.

List the information the mortuary will need to know.

Review "Planning the Funeral" and begin to make arrangements for all the details listed. ______________________________

____

____

____

____

____

____

____

Who will be helping you with the planning and in telling their story? ______________________________

____

____

____

____

____

____

____

Who will make sure that all the arrangements are paid for?

____

____

____

____

____

____

____

____

JOURNAL

Hold something of your loved one's possessions and then just begin to write.

Chapter Thirteen

SAYING GOODBYE

Come to Me all you who are weary and heavy-laden and I will give you rest.

~Jesus

GRIEF AND HEALING

At times, everyone has loss in their lives. Some of these losses have to do with goals that weren't met or relationships that ended. Every loss involves some grief and pain.

The amount of grief one experiences is directly related to the bond that was lost. Other factors have to do with spiritual beliefs, cultural traditions, family relationships, and whether or not the person grieving has support. When there is loss, there is grief and how you grieve will be specific to you and not like anyone else's.

What is normal grief?

A better question is, what is normal for you? Some people and cultures are very open about their grief, wailing and crying publicly. Some people and cultures are very private about their loss, internalizing their pain and grieving privately. There is not a right or wrong way. You have to determine your range of emotions, culture, and standards.

Regardless, grief does have similarities for everyone. Grief comes over you like a wave. You might be feeling okay, strong, and even-keeled only to suddenly feel as if you were knocked off your feet by an enormous wave of grief. The unpredictability of it is very disconcerting.

You can't push through this you must go with it..

Your grieving will take as long as it takes. I wish I could give you a time line, but it is different for everyone. I can tell you that if you don't do the work of grieving, the pain of loss will not go away.

It is okay. It is only temporary. Keep working on the grief, and it will pass. How long you are in grief will depend on several things.

- Are you avoiding or denying your feelings? Stuffing your emotions only means that you are delaying dealing with them and makes grieving longer.
- Do you feel that you have to get over it quickly? Incomplete healing can lead to emotional problems such as depression which won't really go away until you grieve.
- Are you acknowledging your loss, or minimizing it? This can cause you to shut down your heart in order to not feel the pain and this means you won't experience full joy either until you grieve.

- Will you admit your loss, allow yourself to feel it and take as long as necessary to process it? You will heal more quickly by doing so and are on the path back to restoration.

Grieve now or do it later.

You can't get out of grieving. You might be able to stuff your emotions for a time, but they will surface again and probably at a time when you are least prepared to deal with it. Grief waits for you to give it attention and is willing to wait years.

Don't let others tell you how to grieve.

Nor should they tell you what to feel or tell you to pull yourself together. They are not you and don't know what your loss feels like. On the other hand, let those you trust help you process and let you know if they believe you are not coming out of your grief.

This will take time. Give yourself permission to grieve and do what you can, not what you "should".

Platitudes from others.

Understand that they don't know what to say but want to help. So, when you hear, "everything's going to be alright" or "he's in a better place," know the speaker's heart is probably in the right place. A simple "thank you" will do.

EMOTIONAL CHANGES DURING GRIEF

Your emotions may also swing wildly. Laughter and pain can both be part of your grieving reality. You might move from sadness to anger to numbness to tears to an as yet unknown emotion. These swings can make you feel almost as if you are going crazy. This is normal in grieving and a bit scary. Just know that your emotions are going to be erratic.

If you have not lost a loved one before then this depth of hurt might be very new to you. It is almost as if you have entered a different world and can't seem to find a solid path. The pain can feel absolutely crushing and unbearable. I know. It *will* get easier, I promise. Right now, it is so hard. Let it be hard so you can move through it.

Sadness

It goes without saying that you will feel sad, but the level of sadness you feel may be different than you expected. Perhaps you will find that tears come and go throughout your day even when you try to stop them. Your sadness may not result in tears but a feeling that the weight of the world has been placed on your shoulders, and it is even hard to breathe.

Sadness dampers everything and steals your motivation. But it does lessen with time. Be prepared: you can expect twinges of sadness to come unexpectedly even years later as you are reminded of your loved one.

Anger

You may feel anger at God, your loved one, yourself, and/or the world. Death seems so very wrong, and there is nothing you could do to stop it. You might get angry at those who seem to be happy and enjoying life because no one should be happy at a time like this.

Anger is a normal part of grief. Solomon said, "the words of one in grief are like the wind." In other words, we should let the words of strong emotions blow past because they may seem inappropriate or out of proportion. Your grief may cause you to lash out. Realize that it is your heart's pain speaking.

Guilt

It seems that there are many reasons to feel guilty after death. Few of them are legitimate.

Maybe you feel guilty because you are glad it is over and wonder what kind of horrible person would think such a thing. It is perfectly legitimate to be glad that your loved one is not suffering and that this hard journey has ended. Being glad it is over is very common.

You might experience guilt because you think you didn't do enough or what you did wasn't done well enough. Yes, you probably made mistakes, but you are human. No, you were not perfect, but perfection belongs only to God. You did what you could, with the limited skills you had, at a time of great stress and heartache.

You might feel "survivor's guilt." This happens often in an accident where a loved one is killed but another survives. "Why me? Why wasn't it me instead?" The question haunts and accuses.

You are here now because God wants it so. You have done nothing wrong, and you still have much to give this world.

MENTAL CHANGES DURING GRIEF

Grief actually affects your brain and how it functions. The "brain fog" you feel is very real. You become forgetful and distracted and life can feel surreal during this time. This is why it is not good to make any big decisions right now and why it is difficult to make the small ones.

Your cognitive ability might seem greatly lessened as you struggle to concentrate on what people are saying and what is going on around you. This temporary impediment will resolve itself. Your mind will start to clear, your focus will come back, and the fog will recede. Just give it some time.

PHYSICAL SYMPTOMS OF GRIEF

The stress of grief shows itself in physical changes that may become a problem if the grief is extensive. You might experience changes in your appetite and be unable to eat or to eat much. This can be a problem as stress depletes your immune system and makes you vulnerable to illness. Good nutrition is essential at this time. If you can't eat much, eat well.

You may feel a level of exhaustion that makes you unable to function at your normal intensity. When you add in the mental and emotional effects of grief, then you should expect that many activities will take longer than if you weren't grieving and tire you out more quickly.

BEHAVIORAL CHANGES IN GRIEF

Expect to be different from your usual self: you aren't your usual self, after all. You have just lost someone you love. You feel different, your body aches in new ways, and your mind is not thinking clearly. All of this is going to change your behavior somewhat. The differences may be subtle or very obvious. You are moving from who you were to who you will be. What you have been through is life changing, so you can expect behavior changes as well.

Here are a few things you might experience with grief:

- loss of appetite
- inability to sleep
- too much sleep
- dreaming about your loved one
- nightmares
- crying uncontrollably
- joking inappropriately
- being unable to see or be around your loved one's possessions
- having to hold onto a keepsake of your loved one
- withdrawing from the world
- going out into the world almost frantically
- talking to your deceased loved one
- drinking or drug usage
- lashing out in anger
- processing many hours a day
- having no interest in normal activities
- wanting to get back to life and forgetting all of this
- moving closer to God and seeking Him
- needing to talk a lot about your loved one

SOCIAL CHANGES

Grief can make you withdraw from life. You go to the store only to see that life is going on as usual for everyone else, but it has changed dramatically for you. You go through the motions of life, stunned by what has happened.

You might withdraw from a social group of which you have previously been part or join a new group of which you've never been a part. You may have new interests after going through this journey. For instance, you may want to be a support for others who have the same type of journey. Watch your social changes to make sure they are healthy and ask for input from someone you trust if you are not sure.

GETTING STUCK IN GRIEF

The majority of people are able to move through their grief and get back to living their lives. However, some people can't seem to get out of grief. It is certainly not abnormal to feel grief at your loved one not being present at Christmas when they passed in February. Those first holidays and special occasions without them are hard. But I'm talking about something different.

When you are stuck in grief, life feels dark and hopeless. It is hard to see that there could be light at the end of the tunnel. You wonder if you will ever feel normal again. You find that anger or depression has settled in with you and you don't know how to get clear of it.

GETTING OUTSIDE HELP

Hospice provides counseling service for the family for a year after the death because they realize that grief isn't a quick process. They realize that some people can find that they need help months after their loved one has passed. If this is you, then call them. Let them help you.

There are also **grief support groups** that you can join. A group helps you to feel normal because you hear that others experience the same type of thoughts and emotions that you have. They really do know what you are going through and that can be a great comfort. You can support one another as you heal.

Individual and family counseling is another option for healing your grief. Being able to speak one-on-one with a counselor can help get you back into life and out of being stuck in grief. Hospice can provide you with a counselor or refer you to one.

WORK OF GRIEF

You have to do the work of grief if you are to come out the other side. This work is feeling, talking, processing, praying, crying, dealing with your anger, feeling your loss.

It is resting and eating and caring for yourself when you don't feel like it. It is listening to the words you are telling yourself and not allowing your mind to dwell only on the negatives. Your emotions will follow your thoughts. If you feel that you are going to a very dark place, listen to your self-talk. You will find that what you are telling yourself is very dark. You can change that self-talk to be more positive and hopeful and that will help your mood.

One of the best ways to work out your grief is writing and drawing. You can write letters to your loved one and to God. You can just write and write and write and get what is spinning in your mind down on paper. It will be hard but is very much like vomiting: it feels so much better when it is over. You will feel better as you continue to write. You will be actively processing the journey and coming to healing and closure as you take the time to do this.

When you are done writing, feel free to destroy it. The act of doing so helps show you that you are free to move on. Write it down; let it go, start to heal.

SAYING GOODBYE

Goodbye is a continuum not a one-time event. You said this when your loved one passed, and you continue to say it every day. As you move on and do things alone that you used to do with your loved one, you have to say "goodbye" again. With every "first," first birthday, holiday, and special occasion that you celebrate without your loved one there with you, you again say "farewell." There will be many painful reminders that your loved one is not here. With each of them let them go—say "goodbye."

INTEGRATING YOUR LOVED ONE'S LIFE INTO YOURS

At first thinking of your loved one might bring you pain, but as you move through grief—you will be able to look back and revisit your memories of this person.

There is a tendency to whitewash memories of our loved ones who have gone on. At the funeral, most people won't say anything negative about the person even though the deceased may have been an extremely negative person. Don't sugarcoat. Be honest. Tell your story of life with your loved one.

As you review your life with your loved one keep what is best from the relationship—what you learned and loved—and take it with you. Release what was worst in the relationship, giving more forgiveness and letting go of any wrong that was done.

You can change for the better from the good and bad of the relationship. This is what the work of grieving can do for you.

HELPING CHILDREN IN GRIEF

Children grieve differently than adults. Let's start with the fact that they don't always understand it. Young children are used to watching cartoons where characters come back to life or can't die. Older children realize that people do indeed die but never really thought it would happen to someone they knew.

When death comes close to a child, it has also come close to those who would normally help them. These adults are now dealing with their own grief and the details of funerals and phone calls and other responsibilities. The routine of daily childcare that gave the child security may now be gone. So, not only has a loved one passed, but those still here are not always able to be there fully for the child, and that is frightening.

Children need you at a time when you may have little to give. They need to know that they are loved and safe and that it is okay for them to show their emotions.

Children who are struggling act out. This acting out could be showing anger, being irritable, withdrawing, regressing to an earlier childhood state, and other behaviors. They may have nightmares and show fears that they did not have previously. They need help grieving.

When my brother died, my daughter—who was only four at the time—was very angry with him. He had left her a teddy bear, and she said she didn't want it. I helped her to write a letter to him. She told me what to say, and I wrote it. It was short but clear, and when she was done we burned it. She watched the smoke rise to the sky. She knew he had received her message and felt closure. She was able to say her goodbye to him and then retrieved the teddy bear—which she slept with for many years. I was able to grieve and to help my child grieve, as well.

If our emotions are powerful during this time, we also have the resources to deal with them. Children do not. It is imperative that they not be overlooked at this time. It might even be wise to have hospice help if you feel that your child needs more help than you can give.

Remember that teenagers are not adults. Although they have more resources and understanding, they still need your help. They are already going through huge turmoil just being a teen, and this added stress means they do need you. Their support group is usually other teens who also do not have an adult understanding and who are also going through their own turmoil. Don't assume that their friends will be there to help them enough. Watch for any signs that they are not handling their grief well and get help quickly when needed.

FINDING PEACE

In grief, you will be looking for peace. It is that place where you accept your loved one's life, its impact on yours, and accept that for now, you cannot see your loved one. Finding peace ultimately happens when we go to the Lord with our pain and find His comfort. I know you might be angry with Him over the loss of your loved one. That is okay. He understands. His son died once.

I encourage you to go to Him and you will find Him as your comfort and strength in a time when you need both greatly.

CHAPTER THIRTEEN WORKBOOK

What is a special memory you have of your loved one during their life? ______________________________

____
____
____
____
____
____
____
____
____
____
____

What is a special memory you have of your loved one during the journey? ______________________________

____
____
____
____
____
____
____
____
____
____
____

How did your loved one impact your life? ______________________

How will you remember your loved one? ______________________

JOURNAL

While I thought that I was learning how to live, I have been learning how to die.

~Leonardo Da Vinci

What I feel now that you are gone and the journey is over...

Chapter Fourteen

BACK ON SOLID GROUND

Don't ever save anything for a special occasion.
Being alive IS the special occasion.

~Author Unknown

GETTING BACK TO LIFE

Your journey was intense as was the grief after it. But a time does come when life returns to balance. Now, you look back on this time and are able to see it with more perspective.

Doesn't life seem so much more precious and fragile now? Isn't it harder to waste the days you are given? Isn't life itself a miracle and valuable? You cannot walk a loved one to death's door and turn back to your own life unchanged.

SEEING WHO YOU HAVE BECOME

Yes, it was hard, that journey, but it was also amazing. As you look back, you see that being a part of this sacred passage made even the pain worthwhile. You realize that you are stronger, gentler, and more present as a result.

You start having fun and enjoying life again. Isn't this what your loved one would have wanted? You realize that you served your loved one well, even if not perfectly, and it is okay to live again.

Some days you barely think about your loved one. The time span widens between those thoughts. At first, your loved one and the journey were constantly on your mind, but now you are coming back fully into the world physically and mentally. You integrate your loved one's life and its impact on you into your daily life now.

You have changed through this journey, but the life around you kept going on. You may not fit as you did before. It is time to be who you have become as a result of what you have been through.

Your interests may have changed. Perhaps before this you were not so in-tune with eternity and lived more for today. Now, you realize that life is bigger than just the days you will walk the earth. Now you want to live your life more circumspectly. That could mean less focus on acquiring material possessions as you saw first hand that you leave this world without them. Maybe you have a new interest in caring for others and want to change your career to match. Or, maybe, you go back to your normal routine and career but realize that you have more depth to your soul than you did before.

However it manifests itself, you are changed.

FINDING JOY IN YOUR JOURNEY

Watching your loved one die was hard, uncomfortable, frightening, amazing, and transforming. Looking back it is one of the most profound experiences of your life. As difficult as it was, you grew tremendously. Some of that growth was terribly painful to go through. Some of what you discovered in yourself was not who you wanted to be. However, you also found strength you never knew was there. You learned patience and found peace. You are glad you were there overall.

Now, make sure you find joy in the rest of your very own journey. However long you have until it is time for your final passage, decide to live fully. Smell the roses, take time for joy, and, remember, that life is not about the things in it but about the people with whom you share it.

HELPING OTHERS

One more thing, you are uniquely qualified now to come alongside others who are embarking on a similar journey. When you say, "I know how you feel," you actually will. You will understand the stress and the insecurity of the journey, but you will also know how you were able to learn and grow and make that passage and that God really did support you the whole way.

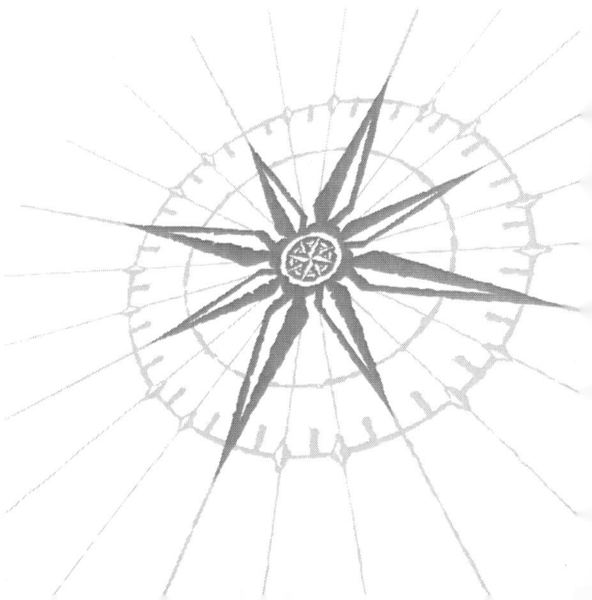

CHAPTER FOURTEEN WORKBOOK

Grief has changed you—how? What is different about you?

How is life different for you now?

When you look back on this passage why are you glad you went?

JOURNAL

This journey has...

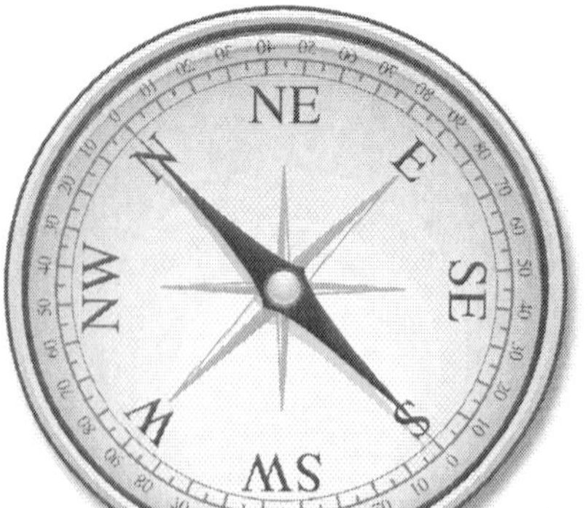
N
NE
E
SE
S
SW
W
NW

Chapter Fifteen

MY PASSAGE WITH MOM

We have two lives—the one we learn with and the life we live after that.
~Bernard Malamud, *The Natural*

The car accident was the first indication anything was wrong. Mom had gone to the store and ended up miles from where she wanted to be. She was lost and had hit another car she claimed she did not see. The hospital staff thought she may have had a small stroke. But the MRI showed a tumor in her brain. Additional tests revealed another tumor on her pancreas and confirmed the cancer in her brain. Both cancers were fatal for a 78-year-old woman.

I drove out from Arizona to southern California. My sister and I were conferring by phone, and I met with some of her doctors. Each doctor wanted to do something different, dependent upon his/her specialty.

Each doctor seemed to be looking only at the tree and missing the forest. I asked each if this was curable. No, but it is treatable. An Internet search about these cancers in elderly people found that length of life was extended by only days to weeks with treatment. That meant we could subject her to radiation, biopsies, drugs, IV's, and considerable pain, and discomfort only to gain a bit of time and lose what quality of life she could have.

I called Mom's general physician to tell him what was going on. He had been her doctor for many years. We spent half an hour on the phone. His suggestion? We should turn to hospice and care for her until she died. I agreed.

We told the doctors at the hospital to stop. We would not torture her until she died. She had 40-80 days left, and we wanted them to be free of procedures and pain and hospitals. We would take care of her.

My cousin Danny and I went to see Mom. She repeated herself often; the brain tumor was beginning to affect her short-term memory. I told her that she had brain and pancreatic cancer, and that it was terminal. Her response was, "Fine. If that is what God wants to do, that is fine with me. My life has always been in His hands and He knows what He is doing." There was no fear, no complaining, just her faith. I told her I wanted her to move to Arizona so I could care for her. She had always said she wouldn't move from California so I was shocked when she was fine with that. I told her I was taking her out of the hospital, and she was elated.

Mom's doctor called hospice, and a man knocked on the door within 2 hours. My sister had flown in, and we sat and talked with him a bit and signed the paperwork. We were both emotional as the reality of what was happening began to take hold.

An intake nurse came that evening to start the process. We told Mom that her doctor ordered home treatment for her since we weren't going to go ahead with biopsies and treatments. Her biggest fear was that there would be "needles." She had a phobia about needles. It was good to tell her that she would never have another in her life.

A CNA was assigned to Mom to help with bathing and dressing. She would come twice a week. A regular nurse would also come twice a week to check on Mom. All medications related to Mom's diagnosis would now be delivered free to our door. Any supplies we would need would also be delivered free. These could include diapers and wipes, hospital bed, and portable potty, wheel chair, walker, etc. Wow. I know Medicare would be charged for this. We had been concerned about all of this, and it was such a relief to have them take care of it.

I left for Arizona to prepare my home for Mom. I'd be back soon to take her from the home she'd lived in for 22 years. I would move her to Arizona to live and die with me.

What better way to transition Mom to our home than to throw a welcome party. We had family and friends over for a barbeque and swim. Mom thoroughly enjoyed herself and ate two hamburgers. I didn't finish one.

The steroids are doing their job. They kept down the swelling in her brain around the tumor and they give her an appetite. Within a day of starting the steroids, we saw a vast improvement in her cognitive ability and loss of confusion. A wonder drug for sure. Before the steroids, it had been hard to get Mom to eat. Now, three meals and chocolate are par for the course.

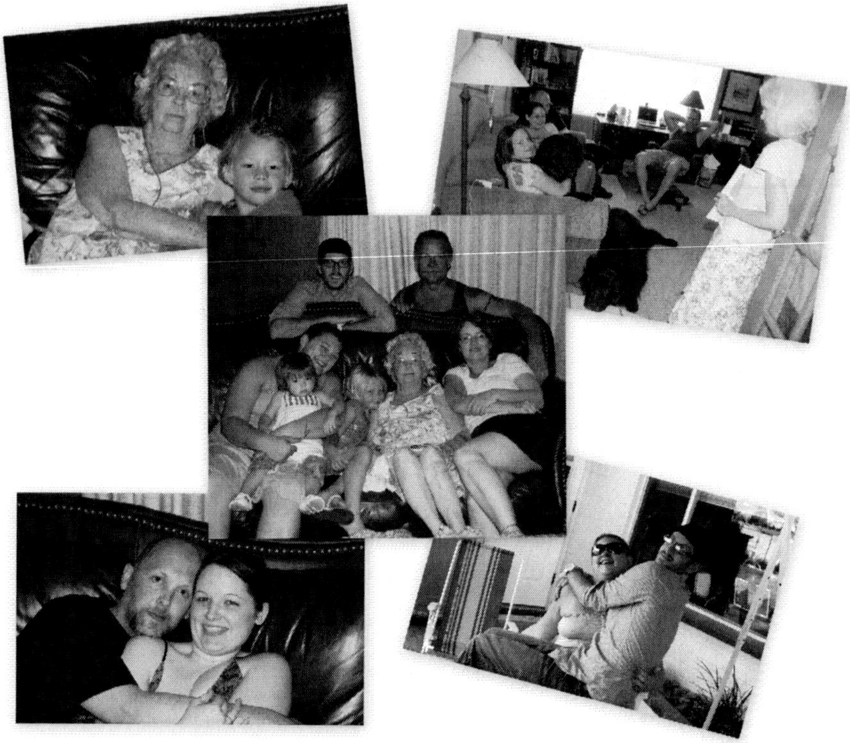

Mom has been here only three weeks and I am exhausted. The endless repetitive questions and the lack of sleep are wearing me down.

I took the dog out to the lawn and just wanted to cry. I'd gotten Mom to bed finally at 11:30 pm and went right away to bed myself. She was up at 6:30 am and, so, I had to be too. I am soooo tired. From the time I get up until I go to bed I'm caring for Mom.

At this stage the care is helping her move around the house, preparing meals and meds, bathing and dressing and coffee, and changing the channel and answering the same question over and over. She watches endless Law & Order *type shows, but doesn't always know what is going on in them.*

I will go to my office to work but am always wondering what she is doing in the back of my mind. Will she try to go outside only to fall and break a hip? Does she need meds or food or…?

Most days I talk with or see someone from Hospice. They are a God-send… and also add to the stress. Nurses or caregivers coming and going need my interaction and input. The dogs have to be put away when they arrive and let out when they leave. I'm tired.

I hate whining. I don't want to whine.

Back out on the lawn this morning, I took a deep breath and did not let tears come forth. Instead, I said, "Good morning, Dad." Then I went on to thank Him for the day. To notice His design of flowers and clouds. To tell Him of my fatigue and my gratefulness for His presence and strength.

The morning could have gone either way. It started going downhill from moment one and when I reached out to my Father, it changed course. I am still so very tired, but my heart is hopeful and I do have joy.

Today I requested a volunteer from Hospice. I need dog food, a few things at Target, and just time alone with God. I need to renew so I can answer the repetitive questions in love rather than aggravation. I need to take care of me so I can take care of her.

Picked up a video monitor today. I love it! From my office I am typing this and watching Mom on the monitor. I used to get up every few minutes and check on her. Now a quick glace and I can see how she is doing. Already I feel a bit of weight lifting.

Burt and I talked about how to manage our lives now. We want to care well for her and for us. We need to ensure that we can still have time alone and that our lives do not become entirely about Mom. We serve her without losing ourselves.

I know there will be that time when most of our minutes are taken up with essential care, but we need to be able to do that based upon the foundation we build now.

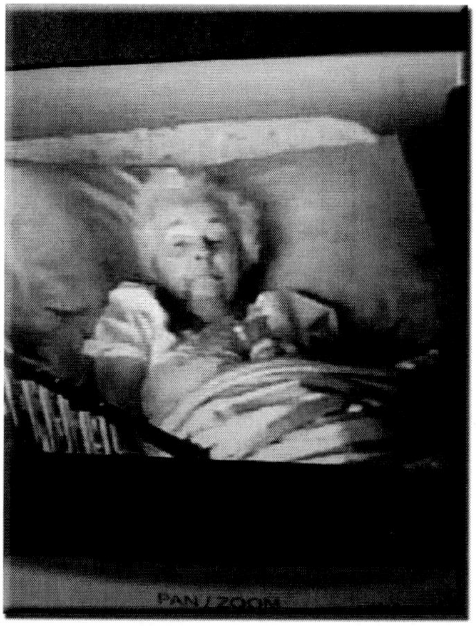

The hospice gave me the names of funeral homes, complete with prices. If I pick the inexpensive one, am I a bad daughter? I guess that is how one spends so much on funeral arrangements—guilt. Spend more and you are a dutiful, loving daughter; spend less and you are disrespectful, ungrateful, and cheap.

Mom had dad cremated and buried in the veterans' cemetery because it was inexpensive. She wants to be cremated and buried next to him. I pretty much dislike this whole process. I am glad I am doing this ahead of time, and that I have a list rather than having to call around after she passes. It still stinks.

I am going to go with the least expensive mortuary and reject the lie that it makes me uncaring. Spending money on her after she dies is not an indication of love and care for her while she is here, and saving money is not an indication of a lack of love today.

Sigh.

I watch her on my little monitor sleeping on the couch as I plan her cremation. My stomach hurts.

The CNA called and said she was on her way to bathe Mom. Since she was still asleep, I figured I better get her up and coffeed. What I found was.... I have no words.

While I was still sleeping, noiselessly Mom had tried to get up to go the bathroom. Her legs were still hanging over the side of the bed and she was lying back asleep. From her waist to knees, her hands, the bed, the carpet, her clothing was covered in excrement. She had some serious diarrhea.

As I walked in the room, the smell hit me. Wow. I woke her and she was pretty out of it. I tried to help her up, but she seemed unable to sit up on her own or hold her weight standing. As I mostly carried her forward, poop was falling off of her. I called for my husband to help, but he didn't hear. I got Mom into the bathroom and seated her sideways on the closed toilet. I ran for my husband, and when I got back Mom, unable to hold herself up, was lying across the toilet and tub. Just then, the CNA arrived. She took over bathing Mom. It was an hour before she was done.

Burt and I spent the next five hours cleaning—the bed, the bedding, the carpet, the floors, the bathroom. Mom, with her short-term memory loss, thankfully remembered none of this.

For the first time since I had heard Mom was dying, I broke down and sobbed. Seeing her like this, so out of it, so weak, so not in control of her body was the trigger that caused all the stress to break forth. The change that had occurred overnight really brought the truth forward: Mom really is dying. Burt, my hero in all of this, just held me and let me cry.

We decided it was time for a hospital bed and bedside potty. They said they could deliver both today. Bringing Mom here to a normal bed rather than a hospital bed felt like we were not telling her that she was coming here to die. We wanted to wait until we reached the stage where we had to have a hospital bed. I just didn't think it would come so quickly.

The delivery man showed us how to operate the bed and the potty. He said that a bit of white vinegar in the bucket would help with the smell, and it does. Amazing little fact.

We set the room up, and Mom came in. She didn't seem too concerned about the change. She is very willing to give up her rights to just about everything. She says, "alright, if that's what you want" or "whatever." It isn't depression, just a letting go of preferences for things that don't really matter. She is letting us care for her.

The potty in the room, which sounds worse than it is, makes a middle of the night got to go session so much easier. I put the potty right next to the bed, help Mom up, turn her to the side, and sit her down. Then I reverse the process when she is done. She is back to bed in minutes.

Friday: The nurse came just as Mom was waking. Mom needed to use the potty, but when I was helping her up she seemed very weak. She seemed well enough but a bit more confused. I helped her down the hallway to the living room, and her left side was still very weak. By the afternoon, she had lost the ability to stand.

My friend, Carrie, came to spend the day with me. Carrie is also a nurse, and she showed me some tricks of the trade. While Mom slept, she taught me to make the bed in layers. That way, if Mom had another accident, I could clean her up, roll the dirty linens up, and a new, clean bed would be ready underneath. That turned out to be a good thing because the next morning, the bed was soaked.

Okay, how did she say to do this? I got a bucket, washcloth, and cleanser and started to clean Mom up. I rolled her to one side, rolled the dirty bedding up like a tortilla then rolled Mom back onto the clean sheets underneath. Then I just continued to remove the dirty ones from the other side. Cool. The waterproof pads I bought kept the new layer clean and dry and had worked well.

Back to Mom's weakness. Mom had to go to the bathroom while in the living room. Because she had walked down the hall earlier, we thought it would be good for her to walk again to the bathroom. When we tried to help her stand, her legs were like cooked spaghetti. She had no strength at all. I ran and brought the potty out and Carrie and I helped her on it. We were both amazed at the change just a couple of hours had brought.

The nurse had suggested it was time for a wheel chair, and it was a good thing. I don't know how we could have moved her back to bed without it.

Kelly, her hubby Terry, and my other daughter, Nikki, flew in to be of help while Burt was out of town. They were astonished at the change in Mom since they had seen her a month earlier. Before they would sit with her and laugh and talk; now she was turned more inward. She no longer initiates conversation and seems distant.

It was hard for them. Seeing her every day made it easier for me, but it was such a brutal change for them—especially Nikki. She tried to sit with her grandmother but would have to get up to cry. Grandma was gone, and she didn't know this dying lady. Mom asked her, "where's your grandmother?" and Nikki could only cry. Nikki stepped up to help in other ways. There is a lot to do with many people in the house, and I totally respect how hard it is for her to spend a lot of one-on-one time with her dying grandmother.

Kelly, the caregiver, did what she does best. She gently cared for her grandmother, bathing and putting medication on the sores on her bottom. I let her take the lead and became her assistant. Kelly has had lots of classes on caregiving and was able to show me a few things. It was nice to take a step back.

Terry just loves to sit with Grandma. He helps her eat and makes sure the meds go in and not on the floor. With his disabled arm, he can't lift her, but his ministry of presence and love goes a long way in caring for her.

We had lots of laughter in the house that week. It filled the nooks and crannies and told death that we neither fear it nor wish to fight it. Love was the biggest force in our house.

The morning they left they said "good-bye" to Mom knowing that they probably won't see her again this side of heaven. There were tears then and again when we dropped them at the airport. At least our good-byes are only temporary.

Today was the first day Mom was bed-bound. I used what I had learned to clean Mom and the bed and then turned on her television. Normally I would help Mom to the living room, but again she was dead weight and it is very hard for me to move her from the bed to the potty—let alone down a hall.

In some ways, it is easier for me to take care of her now. I don't have to worry that she will get up and fall, and she will always be where I left her now. It is easier and harder. Having Mom bed-bound is a giant step toward the end.

I got her coffee (she doesn't finish a cup now) and a piece of toast. I am trying to make sure she eats something. The steroids at first gave her a great appetite but now even they don't help. I can maybe get one meal a day in her.

We fell.

I was supposed to meet a friend at 10 am, and here I was waking at 10 am. I couldn't find her number and felt off-balance and stressed. Mom was just waking and needed to use the potty. I put it next to her bed and lifted her and swung her to the left onto it. She had soaked her diaper, and I cleaned it up and changed the bed pad all the while thinking of Dianne sitting waiting for me. When Mom finished, I was going to move her back to bed but didn't think about what I was doing.

Mom can't hold her own weight now. She can't stand and bear any of her 120 pounds. For me to move her (I weigh not much more than her) I need to reach under her arms and hug her tightly, lift her with my knees on either side of hers, and then move to the side and place her back in bed. I didn't. I don't know where my knees were and when we moved to the side, her left side just gave out. I couldn't hold the weight in my off-balance position, and we started to fall.

I hit the corner of the dresser on my side and again and again on the way down. I was able to place Mom between the bed and dresser, and she wasn't hurt. I called for my husband, and my daughter came in. Mom had no idea we were on the floor. Nikki and I started to pull her up and then my really strong hubby came in and lifted her onto the bed.

I felt sooooo bad and lucky she was unhurt. My side turned a deep purple over the day.

Mom sleeps like a baby—a lot. She is awake now maybe only 2 to 4 hours a day. The video monitor enables me to check in without waking her. The free time is a mixed blessing. I can get more done, but it is a sign that we are getting closer to her death.

Burt and I have more time together. We sit outside by the pool, watch the stars circle the North star, and talk. The monitor is on the table, and I listen to her breathe. Sometimes she stops for what seems an eternity only to start again. Mom is always present with us, even when we are not with her.

Burt, at times, asks me if I should put her in a home. He feels he has no say in whether we do or not. There may come a time when I can't care for her, but I want to as long as I can. I don't want to get a call from some stranger telling me Mom passed and asking what they should do with the body. Yes, this changes our lives, but only for a very short season. I want to care for her until she gets to leave this body and this earth. I feel so privileged to help her transition into the arms of the Lord.

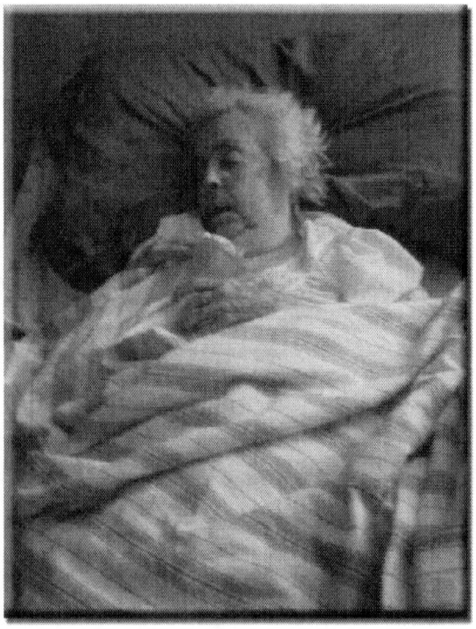

Eating and drinking seem difficult for her now, as is swallowing pills. We have moved to pudding to get pills down. It works well. She likes chocolate the best, and the pills slide right down. She doesn't want to eat more substantial food now, and I give her protein drinks with the pudding —chocolate, of course.

It is all a very messy ordeal. I have to put a kitchen towel under her neck because of the many spills. Sometimes the spoon seems very heavy and she just sets it down on her chest.

Soon I won't be able to get her to take the pills that keep the swelling in her brain and the seizures at bay. This tumor will have its way very soon.

The nurse talked to me the other day about another patient whose daughter wants her on an IV because she is getting dehydrated. We won't be doing that. I will not fight to keep her here; I will not postpone the inevitable and cause her more pain doing so. Mom, with her huge phobia of needles would find it incredibly traumatic. I believe it would pull her out of a coma if she knew she was getting "needles."

We move relentlessly toward her departure and my place in this is to do what I can to help her, not prevent her from leaving.

When Mom first came, it was very stressful. My stomach hurt, and I felt very anxious. Now, I feel peace. My stomach is just fine and anxiety is no longer a constant companion. I think the unknown was a big part of the problem at first. What do I do? How do I take care of her? Will she get up while I'm sleeping and fall? Etc. etc. etc.

Pills and meals and nurses and baths and answering the same questions over and over no longer seem to affect me negatively. I have a sense of something wonderful about to happen. I picture the Lord in the room with her, loving her and about to lift her out of her body.

I have made arrangements for a mortuary to pick up her body when she is done with it. I have an oak container for her ashes that will leave with her when she passes. I read the signs that come at the end of life and see them present. We are nearing the end and I am at peace.

Having the monitor next to my bed reminds me of the days of having a new baby in the house…tuned in to every sound, sleeping but yet listening. Mom's breathing was erratic. She seemed to stop quite often and for what seemed so long a time. And then.....a gasp for air and then minutes of normal breath, only to start the cycle over.

I know there will be a day when that process continues until that next breath does not come. Maybe it is the not knowing if this is the day, if this is the last breath that keeps me from a deep sleep.

Like a baby, Mom is completely dependent upon me. She needs someone to bring her food and drink and help her eat it. She needs diaper changes and to be covered up when cold. She has no capacity to take care of herself. She is helpless.

Like a baby, she doesn't really understand what is going on around her. She recognizes us, loves us and trusts us—but her world is very small now.

The television in her room acts as something to look at. There is movement, sound and color but not a real recognition of what they mean. She no longer can follow the plot of a show or even, at times, know whether the people she sees are real. They seem to be in the room with her, and then they are gone.

I read of others' experience with a dying loved one. I read of long talks and opening dialogue long overdue. That is not my experience with Mom. The brain tumor has demolished her short-term memory and her long-term is fading away. We are left with repetitious questions and answers about eating and where someone is and what I am doing with my day. There is no opportunity for conversations of depth.

On the other hand, I am not dealing with someone in pain and for that I am grateful. But I would love a good talk about what Mom expects when she goes to be with the Lord. About her cherished times in life and those she would love to change. About clearing up those hurts we each gave one another. Instead I answer one more time the same question.

My role with her is mostly caregiving. I change her diapers, bring her pudding with the pills mixed in so she can swallow them. I sit with her and watch the television she does not understand. I agree with her that the color in the painting she does not remember creating is very pretty. I stroke her hair, change her position, apply salve to her bottom.

We never did have a relationship that had a lot of deep conversations. Those times we did surprised me. As children, we don't think of the emotional life and consequences our parents are experiencing. She has let me in on the view from her eyes a few times. It rounds out my own understanding of those days.

The time has passed for us to say those things that I would love to now. All I can do is love her the best I can while she is here.

She tries to tell me something, but I can't understand the slurred words. Her eyes look glassy as if she is not quite in the same world with me.

She has been awake so little today—less than an hour I think. I look at her on the monitor, mouth open, eyes closed and put my ear to the speaker. I wait to hear her breathe. There it is— in, out, in, out. She lives still.

I went in to cover her up and turn out the light. I found myself kissing her on the forehead and saying, "good night, Mommy." I haven't called her that since I was a child. Good night, Mommy. I want you to go and be free of this body and this world, and when you leave the room will be empty. Just the echo of our voices, memories of caring for your aged, dying body. Go, stay. Death IS an enemy but a defeated one. It will be difficult to see her go, but not overwhelmingly so—since I will see her again.

I woke up absolutely exhausted and stayed that way all day. Then I realized that I hadn't taken my own vitamins for several days. In the beginning, I was aware that I had to take care of myself so that I could take care of Mom. Somewhere along the line, I skipped a day and then another and another. I take some really strong vitamins, and they make a huge difference with their presence or absence. It took a couple of days to begin to feel the exhaustion lift.

It seems so near to her death but the days continue to add up. Each morning she is still with us, and every night I turn out the light and close the door as she sleeps. I am in no hurry for her to go but am surprised that she is still here.

Mom doesn't know where she is now and at times thinks I am someone else. As soon as I correct her, she seems to remember me.

Mom was given last rites today. I am not Catholic, but since she is—I knew it would be important to her. The priest asked if she wanted them, and she said she did. I was anxious that she would be scared if asked. She doesn't always know where she is. Being told she is dying if she doesn't remember at that moment could be frightening. But she did know.

It was so hard not to cry. We are finally getting really close. I have been going about the tasks of caring for her: time to change her diaper, time for pills, time for a drink, time for nurses and bathing and…we are out of time.

I watched her mouth move, eyes closed, as she said the Lord's Prayer with Fr. Tony. She received communion and a tear came from her eye. The ritual brought her comfort. There was something holy about it even if I don't agree with the theology.

After he left, I went in to check on her and saw that she was still tearing up. I asked if she needed anything—no. I asked if she was scared—no. I asked her if there was anyone else she wanted to talk with and she said, "only God." I could only cry and tell her how much I was going to miss her.

We talked just a bit about her seeing Dad and Jay and her family soon. I told her that she would see God soon, and she told me she already had. He had told her that she would be home soon for always. I can't remember the exact words.

I realize that although I know she will be free of this body and home soon, I had not been ready to let her go. I thought I was. I would have told you I was, but the last rites released her to go, and I knew I had to let her.

I told the Lord that I let go of her to Him. I released myself to Him disconnected from Mom. We are separating, each going with the Lord at this fork in the road.

After her last rites, she seemed to have permission to go. She started to change that night. The next day she became very restless. "Terminal restlessness," they call it. She seemed in pain or, at the very least, incredibly uncomfortable in her skin. She complained for the first time of pain in her injured arm. I gave her liquid morphine and later liquid Ativan for the anxiety. She seems to have lost the ability to drink, almost as if she has forgotten. She started talking incoherently later in the evening and was unaware of my presence.

This morning she is unconscious. I changed her diaper and the bedding, and she never awoke. I have no way to give her the usual medications but can still give her the liquid ones to help with the restlessness.

I am sitting next to her listening to her struggle to breathe. She has settled down a bit, no longer struggling with her bedding and moving her legs and arms. My daughter and her husband are coming this evening from Seattle. I hope they make it in time to say "goodbye."

Knowing that we are at the end has been surprisingly painful. The transition in the past two days has been dramatic, and the next one will be even more dramatic. In days? hours? She will be gone. She is almost free of this body and this world. I rejoice as I feel this tearing pain in my heart. It is crazy to feel excited for her. I have a deep sense of loss at the same time. I pray and the Lord's presence and peace are here. I remember that He cried before He raised Lazarus. He knows the pain that death causes and calls it an enemy.

I also remember that the sting of death is short and without permanence. We will see each other again. Still, I cry off and on and expect that to continue. I look around her room. I remember preparing it for her, putting her favorite things where she could see them. The Lord prepares a place for her, and it will be perfect and wonderful. All these things I will take down, pack away or give away. What she gets in heaven will be permanent.

I feel as if I am rambling here on the page. How do I write out the ambivalence, pain, joy, apprehension, and relief? There are no words sufficient for such depth of emotion.

Had a melt down. The nurse came by and checked Mom and confirmed that death is imminent but told me it could be days. Mom is so stubborn, and the stubborn ones can hang in there with no food or water or consciousness for up to a week. I have been by her side all day listening to her struggle, thinking she could pass any moment. Last night I didn't sleep and haven't really slept for the past seven weeks. I have been crying a little on and off all day and just couldn't hang in there any more.

I called a friend who had offered meals when Mom first came and told her I needed to take her up on that offer now. Blubbering like an idiot I left her a message and when she called right back I wasn't much better. I am not one who takes help easily. It isn't because I think I'm too good for it or don't need it; I just tend to get things done on my own.

The nurse hugged me and made it harder for me not to cry. I feel weak and stupid and hate this.

Dianne dropped off the food and offered the comfort of her shoulder to cry on. She suggested we go in to see Mom and pray. I was so close to tears and still felt an incredible tenderness toward Mom. I stroked her forehead, and Dianne said she could tell that Mom relaxed a bit under my touch.

We prayed, and Dianne asked that the Lord would take Mom, even tonight. Kelly and Terry were at the airport and on their way here. I so wanted them to make it before she was gone.

I sat alone with her looking at her face and realizing I would see it not much longer. She started to become restless again, and I wanted to wait to give her more morphine just in case she could rouse when they arrived. But I didn't want her to suffer, so I gave it to her.

I heard the car pull up and rushed out to bring them in. It was hard for them to see her but, to my amazement, she roused just a bit and knew they were there. I had told her they were coming and that she had to wait until they arrived. She was unconscious but must have heard. She took a bit of water from the spoon Kelly held. She and Terry sat with Mom and loved her.

We talked a bit, and I said that she might need to hear from them that it was okay for her to go. After I left the room, they both did.

Burt, Kelly, and Terry were in the living room and I sat with Mom. I read 1 Cor 15—"this mortal must put on immortality and this perishable must become imperishable…death where is your sting? It is swallowed up in victory." I talked with her about shedding this old body and becoming all that God designed for her. That she would be beautiful and filled with life. Then I read the last four Psalms. Psalms of praise. This is what you will be doing Mom—soon.

I said my last words to her, asking forgiveness for those days in my youth that I know were hard for her. I told her how much I loved her and that she was free to go.

I had felt the presence of the Lord standing near her bed, and then He leaned over her and her breath stopped. This was different than the other times. I called for the family, and they rushed in. "She has stopped breathing for a long time now." Just then she took another breath and then stopped.

Kelly's hand was over her mouth and Terry teared. Burt stood at the end of the bed watching for each breath. I stroked her head, and told her it was okay.

Kelly had been texting our other daughter asking if she wanted to talk to Mom and quickly called her. She didn't want to just say, oh, sorry, she died. She asked if Nikki wanted to say "goodbye" to Grandma, and she did. She held the phone to her ear and the last words she would have heard was "I love you, Grandma."

One last breath.

We watched. Would there be another? We saw her chest move as if it was trying, but another breath did not come. She was free. She was gone. We cried.

So strange death is. You are here, and then a moment later you are not. I kissed her forehead and said goodbye. I love you, Mom. Thank you so much for letting me care for you here these last weeks.

I walked out of the room to continue talking with my daughter on the phone, who was crying. I was too. So many emotions all happening at the same time. The biggest thing I felt was love.

Mom died surrounded by love. The love of God and her family enveloped her last moments here on earth, and I felt it still present with us. There was grief but hope too that we would be able to share that love with her again one day.

There was a woman named Helen who walked this earth for 78 years. Some of her days, some of her years were not good. Many were focused entirely on herself to the detriment of those around her— much like all of us. But she also blessed many who crossed her path and left her imprint on their lives.

She never fully healed from her childhood wounds, and those disabilities hindered her to the end. She never fully became free in Christ, but there were a few times that she absolutely knew His presence and love. Now, it is her reality forever.

God, in His grace and mercy, brought the two of us together for these few weeks at the end of her life. Somehow, this short time has made up for the years, has been a balm to old injuries and brought us both peace.

It has been my great and amazing blessing to watch her die and help her along this path. Changing her diapers, the feedings and medications, the lost sleep and aching stomach have all been the price paid for the privilege of serving her.

Lord, she is yours now but still my mom. I take joy in the fact that when we meet again, we meet without this flesh but with the glory that you have for us. We will see each other purely, clearly, and perfectly and praise you for the overwhelming honor of walking this road together.

Kelly washed Mom's face after she passed. Mom had problems eating and had a scabby area next to her mouth. It was painful and difficult to clean after she ate. There was a bit of chocolate pudding mixed in with the scabs, and as Kelly wiped it all came off, scabs and pudding. She said she wanted Grandma to be pretty.

It was Jan's job to call everyone when Mom passed. I only had to call her. She thought my job of caring for Mom had to be the hardest, and I thought her job the worst. She made the calls, and I stayed with Mom.

The hospice nurse came and made the call to the funeral home. It would be about an hour, she said. The nurse sat in the chair next to Mom's body, and I stood at the end of the bed. She asked questions and filled out some paperwork. Burt had closed Mom's eyes right after she died and, so, it looked as if she was sleeping. She looked peaceful.

It was very surreal. I recognized my need to talk and let myself do that just a bit with the nurse. I kept looking at Mom's body. So strange that she was not in it. So very odd death is. One moment you are there, and the next you aren't. But you leave behind the container, and it looks like you.

Two men from the funeral home arrived. I said I didn't want to see her taken out in a black bag and was told they don't do that because it is too traumatic for the family. They asked if I wanted her covered or uncovered as they brought her out. I don't know. What a strange question. I've never thought about it. We said covered and then changed our minds. The stretcher was brought in and my son-in-law went into the room with them. He wanted to watch and make sure all was done respectfully. He said it was. They used a sheet to tie her feet and arms to her side. Then they covered her with another sheet and a blanket. When she was brought out, she looked asleep and as if she was just being brought to the hospital. I kissed her forehead and said goodbye; it was cold. We followed the stretcher out to the unmarked, white van and watched them load her. In our family when someone leaves, we wave until we can't see them anymore and, so, we all stood out front waving goodbye until the van turned the corner.

The hospice nurse dumped Mom's meds into a bag of kitty litter and cooked it in the microwave before taking it to the dumpster. She left, and it was just us. It was late now: 1:30 in the morning. Mom had died at 9:58 pm. None of us wanted to go to bed.

I woke with a start. I needed to see what was going on with Mom and what she needed. Oh....she is not here.

My days and nights had been filled with caring for her, and now it was over. I got up and made some tea. I went in her room and looked around. How is it possible that she isn't here?

Burt said that he would take care of stripping the bed and doing the laundry. His quiet and efficient strength are a real support to me.

I feel a bit numb. Because she died Friday night, I have to wait until Monday to go to the funeral home and make further arrangements. I think about her body stored somehow in Mesa. She is still here. Denial says that I can just go there, and she will be okay. All is well, but I do know differently.

We take the day to just hang out together. Some people call. Burt puts the news on his Facebook. He starts to get comments and condolences. Occasionally he reads me a new one, and it is interesting that we are touched by the losses of our friends and family even when we don't know the deceased.

The next day Burt works, and Kelly and I go to Costco. People are milling about, checking their lists, tasting goodies, and living life. Somewhere in the bread section, I start to feel dizzy. A wave of grief almost knocks me off my feet. Life goes on. You are here. You are gone. Life goes on.

Monday we go to the funeral home. There are forms and questions about what we want. I am thankful that Mom had already made those decisions. She wanted to be cremated and buried next to Dad. We had our container already (I'd left it at home) but could bring it after the cremation. There could be almost a week until it happened as the state had to clear that the death wasn't under investigation. No, I didn't want to know when they would do it. Just call me afterwards. They asked if I wanted to see her again. No. Interesting that I could, but she wasn't there. It was just her body, and we had said our goodbyes.
We paid. We left. We waited to hear.

I waited a few days and then asked Kelly to help me clean out Mom's clothes and possessions. She had only moved a few things to my home: pictures, knickknacks, and clothes. I had brought her winter clothes even though she wasn't expected to live that long. Must have been denial.

It seemed early to do this, but I didn't want to do it alone. We wrote out all that we would donate for her taxes, and I was fine until we got to the dresses and nighties she wore each day. I had dressed and undressed her in them, and they seemed to hold all the memories of her stay with me. I put them in the bag reluctantly, carefully, sorrowfully, and pulled the drawstring.

Flowers came, cards arrived, days went by. Kelly and Terry flew home. I started right back to work counseling. Behind my back was the room Mom died in. But life goes on, and these people in my office had pain too. I got the call that I could pick up Mom's remains. Being handed the box and signing the papers was very, very hard. I gave them to Burt and walked out the door crying. We went to lunch. Mom loved to go out to eat.

Sorry Mom, we have to leave you in the car. It's really hot out today, but it was hotter a few days ago for you. Sick humor, but it was so bizarre to have her body in a small box in the back seat that all I could do was make jokes to keep from crying.

At the end of the week, Burt went out of town and I was finally alone.

I woke Saturday and started on a big project. When I moved to doing the dishes, I put a gash in my finger and bolted out to the doctor. The whole time he was putting in the stitches, I was being thankful that this happened when Mom wasn't here. It would have been so hard to take care of her when I couldn't use my right hand anymore.

I went home, took the pain pills as the Novocain wore off, and allowed a few tears to flow down my cheeks. I was sad and tired. I felt dead inside. I missed my mom. This really sucks.

We head to Colorado for a family reunion that had been planned for a year. I love Burt's family and needed to get away. We take three days to drive from Phoenix to Estes Park, stopping one night to sleep and another to visit friends. It is beautiful and fun—and always the grief is with me.

My mother-in-law wants to talk with me about Mom's passing, but I don't want to because I will cry. She is bringing the pain to the surface, and I want to escape it.

We spend another couple of days at Karen and Dave's ranch with our son and his family along, too. It is wonderful, peaceful, beautiful. I am distracted but, still, the grief does not leave. It comes in waves, and I breathe through them. It has only been three weeks after all.

Two days driving home and the waves continue to come. I take about 800 pictures overall and wish I could show them to her when I get home.

Her room is still there. Her box on the shelf. It all comes back in a rush.

Burt and I have dinner outside, and I can't hold back the tears any longer. He didn't realize how hard it had been for me. Guess I am good at keeping this to myself. He tells me that maybe I need not be such a tough girl and sits and listens to me talk and cry. I love that guy.

When he goes in the house, I ask the Lord to come into this place that hurts so badly and He does. I feel His presence and peace, and He seems to take up most of the weight of this load. Until I actually let myself feel it, I couldn't receive His help. By the time Burt returns, I am feeling much better. I have turned a corner in my grief.

That night, I dream of mom. She tells me it is great being where she is. I hug her and she me, and when she is gone—my arms are holding me. I am able to comfort myself. And although I still miss her, we are both okay.

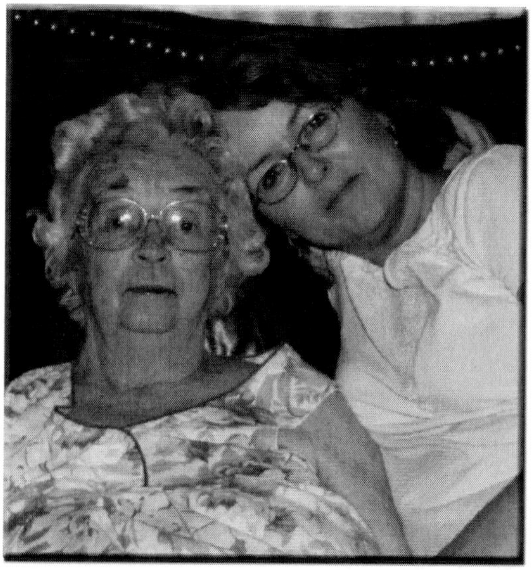

Resources

HOSPICE ORGANIZATIONS

For more information on hospice care and to find a hospice in your area.

National Hospice Organization
www.nhpco.org

National Association for Home Care and Hospice
www.nahc.org

Hospice Foundation of America
www.hospicefoundation.org

HospiceDirectory.org gives listing of every state hospice organization as well as other useful information.
www.hospicedirectory.org/cm/about/state_hospice

ADVANCED DIRECTIVES AND ESTATE PLANNING

Caring Connections provides free advance directives and instructions for every state.
www.caringinfo.org/stateaddownload

ExpertLaw provides information and some free forms to help with estate and power of attorney issues.
www.expertlaw.com/library/estate_planning

MEDICARE BENEFITS

The official U.S. government site for Medicare.
www.medicare.gov

Free website to connect family and friends for the journey
CaringBridge is a 501(c)(3) nonprofit providing free websites that connect family and friends during a serious health event, care and recovery.

A CaringBridge website is personal, private and available 24/7. It helps ease the burden of keeping family and friends informed. The websites are easy to create and use. Authors add health updates and photos to share their story while visitors leave messages of love and support in the guestbook.
www.caringbridge.org

SUPPORT GROUPS

The Compassionate Friends – Grief support after the death of a child.
www.compassionatefriends.org/home.aspx

GriefNet.org is an Internet community of persons dealing with grief, death, and major loss.
www.griefnet.org

CAREGIVING

The Family Caregiver educates supports, empowers and speaks up for the more than 50 million Americans who care for loved ones

with a chronic illness or disability or the frailties of old age.
http://www.thefamilycaregiver.org

Today's Caregiver is a provider of information, support and guidance for family and professional caregivers.
http://www.caregiver.com

Care advice for individuals, families and carers.
http://www.caringinfo.com/

FUNERAL PLANNING

Free consumer information and education resource on funeral planning, financing funerals, funeral products and services, and grief support and counseling.
http://www.funeralplan.com

HOSPICE PATIENTS' BILL OF RIGHTS

Patients have a right to be notified in writing of their rights and obligations before hospice care begins. Consistent with state laws, the patient's family or guardian may exercise the patient's rights when the patient is unable to do so. Hospice organizations have an obligation to protect and promote the rights of their patients, including the following:

Dignity and Respect

Patients and their hospice caregivers have a right to mutual respect and dignity. Hospice staff and volunteers are prohibited from accepting personal gifts and borrowing from patients/families/ primary caregivers.

Patients have the right:

- to have relationships with hospice organizations that are based on honesty and ethical standards of conduct
- to be informed of the procedures they can follow to lodge complaints with the hospice organization about the care that is (or fails to be) furnished and regarding a lack of respect for property
- to know about the disposition of such complaints
- to voice their grievances without fear of discrimination or reprisal for having done so

Decision Making

Patients have the right:

- to be notified in writing of the care that is to be furnished, the types (disciplines) of caregivers who will furnish the care, and the frequency of the services that are proposed to be furnished
- to be advised of any change in the plan of care before the change is made
- to participate in the planning of the care and in planning changes in the care, and to be advised that they have the right to do so

- to refuse services and to be advised of the consequences of refusing care
- to request a change in caregiver without fear of reprisal or discrimination

The hospice organization or the patient's physician may be forced to refer the patient to another source of care if the client's refusal to comply with the plan of care threatens to compromise the provider's commitment to quality care.

Privacy
Patients have the right:

- to confidentiality with regard to information about their health, social and financial circumstances and about what takes place in their home
- to expect the hospice organization to release information only as consistent with its internal policy, required by law or authorized by the client

Financial
Patients have the right:

- to be informed of the extent to which payment may be ex pected from Medicare, Medicaid or any other payor known to the hospice organization
- to be informed of any charges that will not be covered by Medicare
- to be informed of the charges for which the patient may be liable
- to receive this information, orally and in writing, within 15 working days of the date the hospice organization becomes aware of any changes in charges
- to have access, upon request, to all bills for service received, regardless of whether they are paid out-of-pocket or by another party
- to be informed of the hospice's ownership status and its af filiation with any entities to which the patient is referred

Quality of Care
Patients have the right:

- to receive care of the highest quality
- to be admitted by a hospice organization only if it is assured that all necessary palliative and supportive services will be provided to promote the physical, psychological, social and spiritual well-being of the dying patient. An organization with less than optimal resources may, however, admit the patient if a more appropriate hospice organization is not available
    - but only after fully informing the client of its limitations and the lack of suitable alternative arrangements
- to be told what to do in the case of an emergency

The hospice organization shall assure that:

- all medically-related hospice care is provided in accordance with physician's orders and that a plan of care which is developed by the patient's physician and the hospice inter disciplinary group in conjunction with the patient, specifies the services to be provided and their frequency and duration
- all medically-related personal care is provided by an appro priately trained homemaker/home health aide who is supervised by a nurse or other qualified hospice professional

Used with permission - National Association for Home Care & Hospice, 2010
www.nahc.org/haa/attachments/BillOfRights.pdf

Index

About the Author

As you can tell from this book, Kim West has a heart for helping people find healing and make sense of their lives. A Master of Divinity in Counseling and Family and a PhD in Clinical Pastoral Counseling uniquely equip her to care for the heart and the soul. She carries out this mission in her daily life as a Licensed Clinical Pastoral Counselor and Certified Christian Marriage and Family Therapist.

In *Peaceful Passage* she combines her counseling skills with her newly acquired caregiving skills to create a resource that will enable the reader to truly create a peaceful passage for themselves and their loved one.

West lives in Arizona with her husband and has three grown children.

www.peaceful-passage.com

Jacket & Interior Design: ATG Productions, LLC, Christy Moeller-Masel
Interior Typsetting: ATG Productions, LLC, Cory Olson
www.atgproductions.com ~ Surprise, Arizona

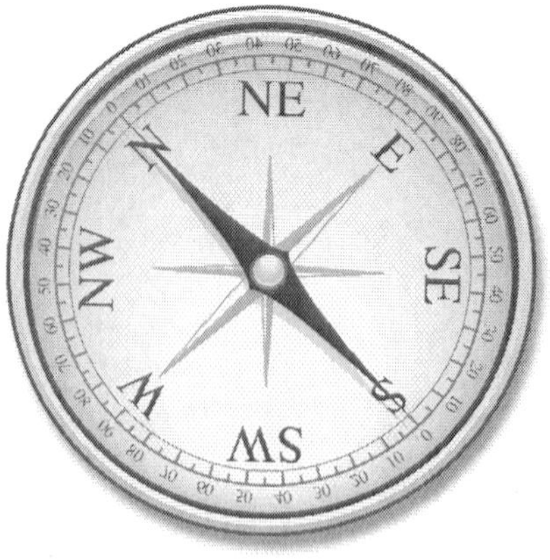